STATINS

MIRACULOUS

OR

MISGUIDED?

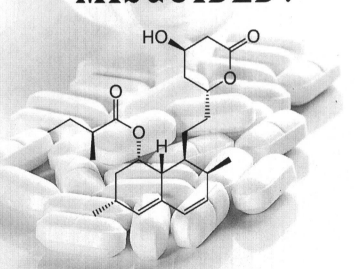

By Mark J. Estren, Ph.D.

RONIN Publishing, Inc.
Berkeley, CA.
roninpub.com

STATINS

MIRACULOUS

MISGUIDED?

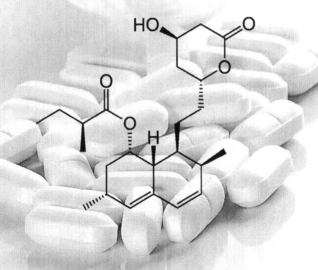

By Mark J. Estren, Ph.D.

Statins: Miraculous or Misquided?
Copyright 2013: Mark J. Estren
ISBN: 978-1-57951-166-1

Published by
Ronin Publishing, Inc.
PO Box 22900
Oakland, CA 94609
www.roninpub.com

Production:
   Cover: Brian Groppe
   Book design: Beverly A. Potter
   Editor: Beverly A. Potter

Credits:
   Illustration on page 14 courtesy National Institute of Diabetes and Digestive and Kidney Diseases
   Photo on page 17 is by Bill Branson, courtesy National Cancer Institute

Library of Congress Card Number: 2013935202
Distributed to the book trade by PGW/Perseus

Acknowledgments

It was my father, Solomon Estren, M.D. (1918-2010), who instilled in me a love of medicine and fascination with the functioning of the human body and the many ways in which its delicate balance is both a wonder and a vulnerability, so easily can it be disturbed. A pioneer in studying the metabolism of vitamin B_{12} and folic acid, translator of Tannhauser's Textbook of Metabolism and Metabolic Disorders, Dad spent more than 50 years in the Division of Hematology and Medical Oncology at The Mount Sinai Medical Center in New York City—and also maintained a thriving private practice in which he was the only doctor. Between being a solo practitioner, making house calls and having a marvelously empathetic bedside manner, he was a complete throwback to an earlier, idealized time of medicine that never really existed. He made it real, though.

He also was co-discoverer of Estren-Dameshek Syndrome, a variation on a rare congenital genetic abnormality called Fanconi's anemia, in which bone marrow does not produce blood cells properly. Many patients with Fanconi's anemia have physical abnormalities such as scoliosis, missing or extra thumbs, a small head and short stature. Some, however, have no physical abnormalities or deformities. They have Estren-Dameshek Syndrome.

Although my early study of medicine did not lead me to a career as a physician—I became a psychology and English Ph.D.—my sense of wonder and excitement about the human body and its functions has never diminished, and as a result, writing about health and medicine has been a prominent part of my life for more decades than I care to count. For all that, Dad, thanks.

Other Books
by Mark J. Estren, Ph.D.

A History of Underground Comics

Question Authority to Think for Yourself

Prescription Drug Abuse

Note for Reader:

The information, analysis and advice in this book
is not intended to replace the services of a physician. This material is provided for informational
purposes only and is not a substitute for professional medical advice. Do not use the information
in this book to diagnose or treat any medical or
health condition or to make any changes in your
medications or other aspects of medical care.
Always consult your doctor and/or other health
professional for any significant issue involving
your health.

Table of Contents

Introduction: The Statin Dilemma 9

1: What Are Statins? 17

2: Lifestyle and Statins 23

3: The Niacin Alternative 31

4: The Natural Approach 41

5: Worst-Case Planning 52

6: The Primary-Prevention Controversy.... 61

7: After a Heart Attack............................ 69

8: The Cholesterol Quandary 77

9: The View from Cleveland 88

10: The Mayo Clinic's View 97

11: Lifestyle with Mayo 104

12: Have a Stronger Heart 112

13: Miraculous and Misguided................. 119

14: The Last Word—for Now 126

15: Furthering Knowledge 132

Bibliography & References....................... 143

Author Bio 149

Ronin Books-for-Independent-Minds 150

Introduction

The Statin Dilemma

Homer Jackson didn't feel quite right. Something was a little off. He was used to the feeling of being overweight, but hey, 205 pounds wasn't all that heavy for a five-foot-nine-inch man. Lots of his friends weighed more. This wasn't a weight thing, though. It wasn't a breathing issue—some of his friends had them, but he didn't. And it certainly wasn't his heart. Homer felt good about his heart. He'd been taking a drug called Zocor®—80 milligrams every day, just as the doctor said he should—and he was careful not to miss a dose. He knew this was a powerful drug, a statin; he'd even Googled its exact name, simvastatin. He knew it was doing its job silently, 24 hours a day, protecting him against heart disease. Several of Homer's friends had already had heart attacks, but Homer was protected. He was 54 and had every intention of sticking around to 94. At least.

But something wasn't right. Homer checked to be sure he hadn't missed a dose of Zocor®—no, he was up to date. He'd missed exercising—well, he didn't really exercise much, so that was nothing new, and that wouldn't explain why he felt so, well, *weak*. His muscles hurt, as if he had in fact been exercising—they were tender. That didn't make sense. He had a desk job. Nothing there to tire him out and make him feel so run-down. Maybe he had a touch of the flu, or something. It would pass.

A week later, it hadn't. Homer was feeling worse. He was tired all the time now, had trouble dragging himself out of bed, wasn't sleeping well even though he kept wanting more sleep. I ought to call the doctor, he thought, but what am I going to say? That I'm tired? Everyone is tired. That I feel weak? Well, I really ought to exercise and build up my stamina—the doctor has told me that before, and I don't want to get into an argument. I'm busy—I don't have time to exercise. And my statin is protecting my heart. Sure, it would be better if I exercised as well, but I'm pretty much okay as is. Just weak.

The muscle pains were worse a week later, and Homer felt stiff and sore all the time. It didn't make any sense at all—he was having the aftereffects of an intense workout without the benefits. And when he went to the bathroom, he saw something else. His urine was a brownish-red color—a lot darker than usual. Not drinking enough, he thought, and started keeping a liter bottle of water at his desk all the time and sipping from it throughout the day.

By a week after that, Homer's co-workers were noticing that he seemed exhausted all the time and was moving as if in pain. His urine color hadn't changed— if anything, it was darker. Homer felt so weak that he could barely function, and he knew it was time to call his doctor, even at the cost of being reprimanded again for not exercising and relying on statins for heart health. He gave in and phoned.

To Homer's surprise, the doctor wanted to see him immediately—the next morning. Now Homer was actually alarmed: it usually took weeks to get an appoint-

ment. He managed to drag himself out of bed and get
to the doctor's office, where he felt like collapsing. And
that's where Homer got the news: his statin, on which he
was relying for a long and healthy life, was killing him.

Statins started, like so many discoveries in medicine,
with something that didn't work. Back in the 1970s,
Japanese microbiologist Akira Endo was searching for
antimicrobials—medicines that would destroy or slow
the growth of disease-causing microorganisms. Endo
was studying a fungus called
Penicillium citrinum, a relative   *Statins started*
of the organism that produces   *with something*
the antibiotic penicillin. He   *that didn't work.*
did not find what he was
looking for—but in a fermentation experiment, he
turned up a natural product with an unusual property:
it prevented normal functioning of an enzyme that the
body uses to produce cholesterol.

Intrigued, Endo called his discovery *compactin* and
set about finding out what it could do. He and other
researchers discovered that it was good at preventing
the liver from making cholesterol, which was already
known to be a factor in heart disease. However, in
higher, more-effective doses, when used longer-term,
Endo's discovery was toxic—it actually killed laboratory
animals. The compound, by now called *mevastatin*, was
never produced commercially, because the risks of using
it, or even testing it in humans, were just too high. This
was the first statin: a dangerous failure discovered when
a scientist was looking for something else.

Good Luck and Bad

Homer Jackson was both lucky and unlucky. He was lucky to live in a time when statins are available. Homer could have brought his cholesterol down through a rigorously followed program of dietary adjustment and exercise, but he had a history of diets not working for him—"yo-yo dieting"—had a sedentary job, and never seemed to find the time to exercise or the willpower to keep doing it, even though he knew he should. Homer was an ideal candidate for statins: young enough to have many more years ahead of him if he could evade the factors making his body a bull's-eye for a heart attack, responsible enough to take medicines prescribed by his doctor on the proper schedule, and not having complicating factors that might have made his doctor think twice about putting him on statins.

Rhabdomyolysis, in which muscles rapidly disintegrate, is a rare but dangerous side effect of statins.

But Homer was in the unlucky 5% of statin users who develop muscle pains from the medicines—pains that can become severe, even debilitating, as they almost did in Homer's case. The American College of Cardiology, the American Heart Association and the National Heart, Lung and Blood Institute all agree that statins are extremely safe in the vast majority of patients receiving them. But not in all patients—and not in Homer's case.

Yet Homer was lucky that he contacted his doctor when he did. Things could have been worse, much worse, if he had waited longer. The generalized muscle pain that Homer experienced could have turned into *rhabdomyolysis*—a condition in which muscles rapidly disintegrate. Rhabdomyolysis is usually due to an injury, such as physical trauma from an accident. But it is also a side effect of statins—and when it occurs, it can be fatal. Homer could have gone into acute renal failure when myoglobin from his deteriorating muscles overloaded his kidneys and caused them to stop working. In fact, one statin, Baycol®, was taken off the market in 2001 after dozens of people died from rhabdomyolysis that was associated with it.

A Fatal Case

Jenny Pearson wasn't so lucky. The 82-year-old Kansas widow had taken a statin for years to control her cholesterol—which it did. She had also had years of muscle pain, which neither she nor her doctor attributed to the statin. Her pains got so bad that Jenny could barely use her shoulder, and ended up having surgery—which did nothing. Jenny later developed skin lesions that looked like a fungal infection, so she was treated with an antifungal drug—which was ineffective, because it was the statin that caused the lesions: they were a result of the muscle breakdown produced by the drug.

And antifungals can significantly increase the risk and severity of statin-caused muscle disorders. Within three months of starting the antifungal therapy, Jenny's condition worsened: she became so weak that she could not stand or breathe on her own. Two weeks later, she was dead.

Homer's luck held in several ways. First, by getting to his doctor before rhabdomyolysis set in, he avoided one of the most serious side effects of statins. Second, it turned out that he did not need the 80 milligrams of

Zocor® he had been taking. His doctor switched him to a different statin at a lower dose—and Homer still got good cholesterol-lowering results. And third, the whole experience scared Homer enough to encourage him to take other actions to reduce cholesterol and improve his general health. Those irritating, inconvenient ideas about changing his eating habits and exercising regularly didn't seem so troublesome anymore—not after he became so weak that he could barely function, and understood that, had he not gotten follow-up treatment in time, he could have died.

A Life in Science

Akira Endo was also both lucky and unlucky. Endo, born in 1933, spent more than 20 years working at chemical company Sankyo, focusing initially on using fungal enzymes to process fruit juice. Endo was good at his job— so good that he won Japan's Young Investigator Award in agricultural chemistry in 1966. His success made it possible for him to spend two years as a research associate at Albert Einstein College of Medicine, and that was where he started working on cholesterol—not as a human problem but in connection with fungi, in which he had a strong interest since childhood.

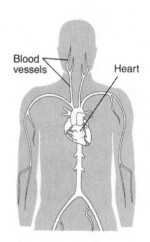

Blood vessels

Heart

Endo knew that *ergosterol* is a component of fungal cell membranes and that cholesterol is needed for manufacturing ergosterol. This led him to study how fungi defeat parasitic organisms. His idea was that the fungi used chemicals to stop or slow cholesterol synthesis.

Like Thomas Edison meticulously experimenting with 10,000 potential light-bulb filaments and discovering that none of them worked, Endo studied 6,000 chemical compounds in searching for ones that fungi might use to inhibit the synthesis of cholesterol. He eventually found three from *Penicillium citrinum* that had the effect he was looking for. One turned out to be compactin—later known as mevastatin.

Endo's luck—and his persistence—brought him multiple awards in later life, including the Japan Prize in 2006 and the prestigious Lasker Award for clinical medical research in 2008.

But he was not lucky in all respects—certainly not in monetary terms. Despite discovering what would become one of the most widely used medicines in the world, Endo, aside from dutifully collecting his salary, never benefited financially from statins at all.

1

What Are Statins?

I t all starts with cholesterol—or rather with the 37-step process by which the body's cells make cholesterol from simpler molecules. Cholesterol has gotten a bad reputation because of its association with heart disease, but without it, animal life would be impossible. Cholesterol is essential to cell structure, being needed to establish proper permeability of cell membranes—that is, to make sure that substances that need to go in are able to, and substances that need to be removed can be pushed out.

Cholesterol is also needed for the body to be able to synthesize steroid hormones, vitamin D and bile acids, which make it possible to process dietary fat. In fact, the word *cholesterol* ties directly to this digestive function: it comes from the Greek *chole*, which means bile, plus *stereos*, which means solid, plus the suffix *ol*, which indicates an alcohol. Cholesterol was first identified in gallstones in about 1758 by François Poulletier de la Salle, a French chemist who lived from 1719 to 1788, but his work was not published.

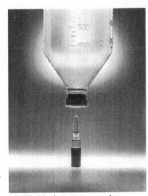

Medicine containers.

It was another French chemist, Michel Eugène Chevreul,

who lived from 1786 to 1889 and was a specialist in fatty acids, who named the compound "cholesterine" in 1815.

Cholesterol is more than important for human health—it is necessary. It is in fact the principal sterol synthesized by animals, and human breast milk contains significant quantities of it. The problem is not cholesterol but *too much* cholesterol: high levels have been linked to damage to arteries and thus to cardiovascular disease.

Dietary cholesterol is not the factor in illness that most people believe.

How much cholesterol does the human body contain? One of the most amazing things about the normal functional balance of our bodies is how small an amount of any given substance is crucial for health, or capable of damaging it. A 150-pound person synthesizes about 1,000 milligrams of cholesterol a day—that is, one gram, which is about four one-hundredths of an ounce. The total body content is about 35 grams, or about one-and-a-quarter ounces. That's it.

In the United States, additional daily intake of cholesterol—from egg yolks, cheese, beef, pork, poultry, fish, shrimp and other sources—averages 200 to 300 milligrams, which is less than one one-hundredth of an ounce. And despite all the attention given to cholesterol consumption, dietary cholesterol is not the factor in illness that most people believe. The reason is that most of it is *esterified,* which means it has undergone a chemical transformation that results in poor absorption—with the result that cholesterol taken in from food has minimal effect on the body's cholesterol content or the concentration of cholesterol in the blood. In fact, the body responds to a higher intake of cholesterol from food by slowing its own cholesterol production, so there is a rather elegant self-balancing mechanism involved in cholesterol synthesis.

So the problem of high cholesterol is not one of people eating too many cholesterol-containing foods—although there are other health reasons for reducing consumption of some such foods. The problem is one of the body itself making too much of this crucial substance.

That is where statins come in. Go back to that 37-step process. It all starts with an enzyme with a mouthful of a name: *3-hydroxy-3-methyl-glutaryl-CoA reductase.* It is sometimes called HMGCR, which is a mouthful of an acronym. Most often, though, it is referred to as *HMG-CoA reductase.* It is a rate-controlling enzyme that affects a particular part of the body's metabolism—the part that produces cholesterol and certain other compounds called *isoprenoids* or *turpenoids.*

Statins target HMG-CoA reductase. The enzyme is central to the production of cholesterol in the liver, where about 75% of the body's cholesterol manufacturing occurs. HMG-CoA reductase contains, logically enough, HMG-CoA—and statins are molecularly very similar to HMG-CoA. Therefore, they take the place of HMG-CoA in the enzyme and reduce the rate at which it is able to produce the next molecule in the sequence that leads to cholesterol, which is called *mevalonate.* Less production of this molecule means, ultimately, less creation of cholesterol.

HDL is called "good" cholesterol and LDL is called "bad," but neither one is cholesterol at all.

All statins, whether naturally occurring or synthetic, work essentially the same way. By inhibiting HMG-

CoA reductase, they block the pathway for synthesizing cholesterol in the liver. When the liver can no longer produce cholesterol, levels of cholesterol in the blood decline.

How Statins are Used

It is the way statins go after HMG-CoA reductase that determines how the medicines are used. Cholesterol synthesis seems to occur mostly at night, so short-acting statins are usually taken at bedtime for maximum effect. Long-acting statins can be taken anytime with no significant difference in their effectiveness.

One reason statins are so attractive for preventing and treating cardiovascular disease is that they go beyond slowing production of cholesterol. They also get at the way in which cholesterol is transported around the bloodstream. This is where HDL and LDL come in. HDL, or high-density lipoprotein, and LDL, or low-density lipoprotein, are the two best-known of the five substances that carry cholesterol to specific tissues. The others are chylomicrons; very-low-density lipoprotein, VLDL; and intermediate-density lipoprotein, IDL. HDL is commonly referred to as "good" cholesterol and LDL as "bad" cholesterol, even though in fact neither one is cholesterol at all: they are cholesterol *carriers*, and the cholesterol within them is identical.

Statins change the balance of LDL and HDL in ways favorable to health. LDL is the major carrier of cholesterol in the blood—one molecule contains about 1,500 molecules of cholesterol in esterified form. LDL gets the cholesterol into cells, where an enzyme makes the cholesterol available for use or storage. But when cells contain enough cholesterol for metabolic purposes,

they will not allow any additional LDL inside—so LDL
molecules stay in the blood
and are oxidized. At that
point, the body's immune sys-
tem goes after them, and protective cells, *macrophages*,
engulf them.

*Statins can even
help people with-
out a history of
cardiac disease.*

So far, so good—but then the filled macrophages
become *foam cells*, and this is where problems begin.
Foam cells are not dangerous as such, but when they
accumulate at a particular place, they create an area of
atherosclerosis—thickening of an artery wall. This becomes a chronic inflammatory response unless the cholesterol is pulled out of the macrophages by HDL and
recycled. If the balance of HDL and LDL is off, HDL
cannot clean up blood vessels efficiently, inflammation
increases, and there is a heightened risk of stroke and
heart attack. This is why, colloquially, HDL is "good"
cholesterol and LDL is "bad."

What Statins Do

In terms of statins, what matters is that the medicines
pull both LDL and VLDL out of circulation, sending
them to the liver, where the cholesterol is reprocessed
into bile salts that are then excreted. At the same time,
statins raise HDL to a modest degree. Result: more
HDL, less LDL, and a better ratio between the two—a
recipe for a healthier cardiovascular system.

The power of statins to rebalance the cardiovascular
system should not be underrated. They even seem to
have benefit for people with no history of high cholesterol: research called the JUPITER study, whose
acronym stands for Justification for the Use of Statins

in Primary Prevention: An Intervention Trial Evaluating Rosuvastatin, found fewer strokes, heart attacks and surgeries for patients who had no history of high cholesterol or heart disease—but did have elevated levels of C-reactive protein, a measure of inflammation.

So, in summary, statins reduce the amount of cholesterol made by the body, and it is that amount—not the amount from foods—that is the major cholesterol supply. Statins work by blocking a specific metabolic pathway, and they do this so efficiently that they not only reduce total cholesterol but also change the balance of the lipoproteins that move cholesterol around the body: they increase the beneficial ones, decrease the troublesome ones, and improve the ratio between the two. Furthermore, statins are so powerful that they can even be beneficial for people without a history of high cholesterol or cardiac disease.

By pretty much any definition, these deserve to be called miracle drugs. What's not to like? The answer, unfortunately, is: quite a few things.

2

Lifestyle & Statins

About 25% of Americans ages 45 and up take statins. This is not really a surprise, given the fact that heart disease is the nation's No. 1 killer for all groups except Hispanics, for whom cancer is No. 1 and heart disease No. 2. Most people can lower heart-disease risk factors without taking any medicines at all, by adopting a more healthful diet, getting regular exercise and losing weight. But these things are *hard*, and while they can lower risk to a certain extent, they cannot necessarily do so to the extent that doctors believe necessary in order to protect the aging cardiovascular system.

Taking a pill, even for the rest of your life, seems comparatively easy. Furthermore, it takes doctors far less time to prescribe a medication than to take patients through multiple counseling sessions on lifestyle changes, including followups to be sure the patients are doing what they say they will do—and the way medical reimbursement is handled by the insurance industry and government is such that those multiple counseling sessions may not be paid for at all, or may be paid for at such low rates that they are not worthwhile for doctors. So factors both personal, involving people's difficulty making lifestyle changes, and financial, involving incentives to see more patients for less time, not fewer ones for longer appointments, combine to make the prescribing of statins highly attractive for patients and practitioners alike.

But this situation comes at a cost. It is not a particularly high financial cost: generic statins cost only about $4 per month, and Stephen R. Smith, MD, MPH, professor emeritus of family medicine and former associate dean of the Warren Alpert Medical School of Brown University in Providence, Rhode Island, says 75% to 80% of patients can achieve the recommended levels of LDL cholesterol—usually below 130 mg/dL is suggested—with generic statins.

However, the use of statins has costs that go beyond their out-of-pocket price. Like any potent medicine, statins do more to the body than what they are specifically intended to do. Muscle pain, digestive problems and potential liver damage are among the best-known side effects.

And then there are costs that statin users may not realize. Yunsheng Ma, MD, PhD, MPH, an associate professor in the division of preventive and behavioral medicine at the University of Massachusetts Medical School in Worcester, coauthored an analysis of statin studies for *Archives of Internal Medicine* in which he found that the drugs significantly increase the risk of diabetes. The studies that Ma looked at included 153,840 postmenopausal women ages 50 to 79, none of whom had diabetes at the start of the study. The women were tracked for an average of 7.6 years, during which time 10,242, or nearly 7% of them, developed diabetes. Even after researchers adjusted for other diabetes risk factors—such as age, race, diet, physical activity level, smoking, high blood pressure and a family history of diabetes—women who took

Mevastatin

statins were 48% *more likely* to develop diabetes during the course of the studies than those who did not take statins. And *all* types of statins had this effect, regardless of the dosage, potency or how long the medication was used.

This is, to say the least, troubling. Patients and doctors alike naturally expect that side effects will be, to a great extent, dosage-dependent—take more of a medicine and the chance of side effects is greater. But not, apparently, when it comes to diabetes and statins—at least in the case of postmenopausal women.

No Reason to Panic

This is not a reason to panic or even a reason to stop taking statins; it is simply a wakeup call for statin users—men as well as women—to understand that statins, like all medicines, have risks as well as benefits. What is an appropriate response to the finding about diabetes? The best thing to do is to talk to your doctor about ways to reduce your need for the drug—which will take you right back to talking about lifestyle issues such as weight loss and dietary changes; discuss an appropriate schedule for screening for diabetes; and immediately alert your doctor if you develop any possible warning signs of diabetes, such as increased thirst, increased urination and/or blurred vision.

The risk-vs.-benefit equation is one to which doctors and patients alike need to pay more attention. It applies as well to one of statins' better-known side effects: fatigue. In another issue of *Archives of Internal Medicine*, Beatrice A. Golomb, MD, PhD, a professor of medicine at the University of California, San Diego, School of Medicine, wrote a research letter on the fatigue issue, interpreting elements of a study of statins' effects on thinking, mood and behavior. The study involved 1,016 generally healthy adults who had moderately elevated levels of LDL cholesterol, but no heart disease or diabetes. Participants were randomly assigned to take either a placebo or a standard and relatively low dose of a statin: *simvastatin* (Zocor ®) at 20 mg or *pravastatin* (Pravachol ®) at 40 mg.

This was a so-called double-blind study, considered the gold standard in medical research: the capsules, which patients took daily for six months, looked identical, and neither the participants nor the researchers knew during the study which group was receiving which treatment—in other words, patients and researchers alike were "blind" to who was getting what; hence "double-blind." At the end of the study, participants reported how much energy they had, comparing how they felt after six months on the pills with how they had felt at the start of the study. They used a five-point scale ranging from "much less" to "much more" to rate their energy level and degree of *exertional fatigue*—that is, fatigue associated with moving around, for example when doing exercise.

The risk-vs.-benefit equation is one to which doctors and patients alike need to pay more attention.

What the researchers found was that statin users were much more likely than placebo users to experience a decrease in energy, worsened exertional fatigue, or both. The side effects were significantly greater in women than men: among female simvastatin users, 40% experienced one of the two types of energy loss, while 20% reported both types.

There are always uncertainties associated with scientific studies, of course, and this one was no exception. The feelings of lower energy were self-reported, which means they were subjective, and some people are more likely to report reduced energy than others. Furthermore, to the extent that the energy decrease was statin-related, there was a distinct tradeoff in the drugs' risks vs. benefits: side effects were somewhat worse with simvastatin

Statin users are much more likely to experience a decrease in energy.

than with pravastatin—but on the other hand, simvastatin was more effective at reducing cholesterol.

And what does this all mean? Well, statins are potent drugs, and generalized fatigue is a systemic reaction, so perhaps statins have an overall negative effect on cell health—after all, they have a full-body effect on cholesterol levels, and cholesterol moves in and out of cells, so it is logical that the medicines may have effects beyond their intended ones.

Stay Alert

But while scientists try to figure such things out and plan additional research, the more important question for statin users is what to do about these findings. The first response should be to stay alert about your own energy level. Plenty of things besides statins can make people feel enervated—life is complicated and stressful enough to sap most people's energy every once in a while. But if you find that your energy is *consistently* lower than it used to be, especially as time goes on and you remain on statins for a longer period, you may suspect that statins are playing a role in how you feel. In that case, request that your doctor factor in your fatigue when gauging the drug's benefits vs. its risks. This is particularly important for patients for whom statins have not been shown to prolong life, including women, people without heart disease, and people over age 70—even ones who do have heart disease. Simply ask your doctor whether you can reduce your statin dosage or switch to a different medication to see if your side effects lessen; this is usually easy to do.

Also—to return to lifestyle issues—find out whether your doctor thinks you could obtain as much systemic benefit from dietary changes, added exercise and weight loss as from statins; but do not be naïve about this, since your doctor may strongly recommend such lifestyle changes, but it will be up to you to implement them. If you go off statins and do not make the changes, you will be responsible for increasing your own cardiovascular risks—and risk reduction is what statins are all about.

Your doctor will likely point out that a better food-and-exercise regimen will not only eliminate any statin-related fatigue but also, in and of itself, give you more energy. But while this is certainly true, it will work only if you commit to the lifestyle changes and follow through on them consistently. After all, your doctor will not be there to supervise your behavior—and for many people, taking a daily pill is simply easier than making large-scale changes in everyday life, even if the medicine comes with a downside, such as fatigue.

What to Watch For

There are additional potential downsides, though, and patients need to take all of them into account when deciding what to do about statins. Years after statins became widely available, the U.S. Food and Drug Administration added several new safety warnings to this class of medicines. Amy G. Egan, MD, MPH, deputy director for safety in the division of metabolism and endocrinology products of the FDA.

New Safety Warnings

- Increased risk of cognition problems such as forgetfulness, confusion and memory loss.

- Elevated blood sugar, especially in people who were already insulin resistant or prediabetic. This ties into the side effect of actually developing diabetes.

- Higher risk for muscle damage when taking certain medicines in addition to statins. For example, medications that can interact with *lovastatin* (Mevacor®) and increase this risk include HIV protease inhibitors, the commonly used antibiotics *erythromycin* and *clarithromycin*, the antidepressant nefazodone, and certain antifungal and hepatitis drugs.

But sometimes when the FDA adds concerns, it also takes some away—or seems to. This constant back-and-forth is an ongoing source of frustration for patients and, for that matter, for health practitioners; but it is simply a fact of life, since the positive and negative effects of medicines become clearer only as they are used by more people for a longer period of time. Thus, when it announced the new warnings, the FDA also dropped one of its earlier recommendations: that patients using statins have routine blood tests to monitor liver enzymes. This seemed like good news for patients, reducing the inconvenience of regular testing and indicating that concerns about statins' effect on the liver were overblown. But not so fast: in fact, the FDA said the reason for stopping the recommendation of regular tests was that the tests did not effectively predict who

The positive and negative effects of medicines become clearer only as they are used by more people for a longer period of time.

would suffer from the rare instances of liver damage associated with statin use. Instead of the regular tests, the FDA said a liver enzyme test should be done just once—before statin treatment begins—and repeated only if a patient should start to experience symptoms of liver damage, such as upper-right abdominal discomfort, dark urine or yellowing of the skin or eyes.

Dr. Egan said patients should simply be more watchful in light of the FDA's warnings, being on the lookout for symptoms of any possible problems: forgetfulness, confusion, excessive thirst or urination, muscle aches or weakness that slow you down and do not seem to get better, or the symptoms of possible liver damage. But this is a lot for patients to think about and watch for, especially when added to all the other things they are also supposed to think about and watch for—not to mention all the symptoms that may be associated with other medicines they are taking, or simply with everyday life stresses.

Suddenly the simple notion of taking a statin pill and protecting your heart doesn't seem so simple anymore. But...hmmm...what about a *different* pill?

3

The Niacin Alternative

Tom Lehrer, a songwriter and satirist famous from the 1950s through the 1970s for skewering social, political and intellectual pretensions, wrote in "I Wanna Go Back to Dixie," a song in which he sarcastically imagined former Southerners idolizing their birth region, "I'll go back to the Swanee—Where pellagra makes you scrawny." The line is funny, but the illness is not. Among its symptoms are high sunlight sensitivity, dermatitis, skin lesions, weakness, insomnia, gastrointestinal disturbance, paralysis of the extremities, and an enlarged and weakened heart, known as *dilated cardiomyopathy*.

The psychological symptoms include aggression, mental confusion, psychosensory disturbances, such as odors causing nausea and vomiting, and psychomotor disturbances, such as constant tension and restlessness. It has been called a disease of the four D's: diarrhea, dermatitis, dementia and death.

Although little known in developed countries to-day, pellagra was an epidemic disease in the American South in the early 1900s, with 100,000 Southerners known to be affected in the 1910s. Scientists believed the disease was caused by a germ or toxin in corn, and the Spartanburg Pellagra Hospital in South Carolina, established in 1914, was dedicated to discovering the cause of the illness.

Joseph Goldberger, MD, a United States Public Health Service epidemiologist who lived from 1874 to 1929, showed in 1915 that pellagra was linked to diet, using prisoners as guinea pigs for his experiments. By 1926, Goldberger had discovered that a balanced diet or consumption of a small amount of brewer's yeast prevented pellagra: he induced the disease in prisoners, with seven of his 11 subjects contracting it, and he then cured them by feeding them fruits and vegetables—after which he was allowed to give them their freedom.

Goldberger did not, however, identify the specific cause of pellagra before his own death, from cancer. It was Conrad Elvehjem, an American biochemist who lived from 1901 to 1962, who, in 1937, identified a previously unknown molecule in fresh meat and yeast that he called nicotinic acid—and showed that this substance cured pellagra. Now we know it as vitamin B-3 or, more commonly, niacin.

Niacin, a colorless, water-soluble solid, is one of only five vitamins that, when lacking in the human diet, are associated with pandemic deficiency diseases; the others are vitamin C, associated with scurvy; thiamine or vitamin B-1, with beriberi; vitamin D, with rickets; and vitamin A, with night blindness. The only grain low in digestible niacin is corn, which is why pellagra and high levels of corn consumption were correctly associated for many years, although the reason for the relationship long remained unknown.

Niacin is one of only five vitamins that, when lacking in the human diet, are associated with pandemic deficiency diseases.

The recommended daily allowance of niacin is 2-12 mg/day for children, 14 mg/day for women, 16 mg/day for men, and 18 mg/day for pregnant or breast-feeding women; levels above 35 mg/day can cause flushing and other side effects, so 35 mg/day is generally considered the tolerable upper limit of niacin intake. But there is an exception to this: much higher daily doses of niacin can be used to promote cardiovascular health—as an alternative or, sometimes, a supplement to statins.

Niacin binds to and stimulates a specific protein receptor called GPR109A. Normally, this receptor prevents the breakdown of adipose tissue—that is, fat. When fat breaks down, lipids are liberated from the tissue and used to build very-low-density lipoproteins or VLDL in the liver. VLDL is a precursor of LDL, which is known as "bad" cholesterol, even though it is not cholesterol at all but a cholesterol transporter. So when niacin binds to GPR109A, it blocks the breakdown of fats—which means there

Niacin

are fewer fatty acids in the blood—which means there is less secretion of VLDL and cholesterol by the liver. And by lowering VLDL levels, niacin raises the level of HDL, which is known as "good" cholesterol—another misnomer. And there you have it: a totally different mechanism for improving cardiovascular factors from the one used by statins.

Downside of Niacin

Niacin has actually been used for more than half a century to raise HDL levels. Why not continue to use it instead of prescribing statins? Well, as with every substance affecting our finely tuned and closely inter-related bodily systems, there is a catch; in niacin's case, several catches. Pharmacological doses of niacin are generally 1.5 to 3 grams per day, and sometimes up to 6 grams—far above what is usually considered the tolerable upper limit. Therefore, side effects of therapeutic niacin are quite widespread. They include skin flushing, itching, dry skin, skin rashes—niacin makes eczema worse—plus indigestion, nausea, liver toxicity, the irregular heartbeat known as cardiac arrhythmia, and elevation of blood sugar. And high doses of niacin cause birth defects in laboratory animals.

Side effects of therapeutic niacin are quite widespread.

Some of these side effects are comparatively rare, but flushing is not—it is so common that it can scarcely be called a side effect at all, and is better described as a primary effect of high niacin intake. And patients find it very annoying indeed. It generally lasts 15 to 30 minutes and sometimes comes accompanied by a prickly or itching sensation, especially in areas of the body covered by clothing. The effect can be lessened by taking one full-dose aspirin tablet half an hour before taking niacin—but that significantly complicates a patient's medication regimen.

A daily tablet of ibuprofen (Motrin®) or naproxen (Aleve®), taken an hour before the niacin, also reduces flushing, but also at the cost of a more-complex medication schedule; taking niacin with meals can help; and taking niacin at the same time as a medication called *laropiprant* can also reduce flushing. The good news is that after several weeks—or sometimes more—of a consistent dose of niacin, flushing disappears or significantly diminishes in most patients. The bad news is that this does not happen in *all* patients, and the extent to which flushing and itching diminish varies widely.

Extended-release niacin, made by Abbott Laboratories and sold as *Niaspan*®, does significantly lower the incidence of flushing. But it costs a great deal more than ordinary, generic niacin, and comes with issues of its own: doses above 2 grams per day of slow-release niacin are associated with liver damage.

Flushing from niacin is so common that it can scarcely be called a side effect at all.

Of course, statins are scarcely perfect themselves. And niacin has some distinct advantages over statins. Steven Nissen, MD, chairman of the Robert and Suzanne Tomsich Department of Cardiovascular Medicine at the Cleveland Clinic, points out that niacin not only increases HDL by 15% to 35% but also slightly lowers LDL, by about 10% to 12%—and reduces levels of *triglycerides*, blood fats that have been loosely linked to heart disease. Furthermore, unlike statins, niacin is naturally present in foods, including meats, leafy vegetables, legumes and whole grains.

Generally, the risk-vs.-benefit ratio of niacin is such that it is recommended for patients with low HDL who are at moderate risk for heart disease and who do not need statins' power to lower LDL. For example, according to Nissen, men with an HDL level substantially below 40 mg/dL—milligrams per deciliter—and women with an HDL below 45 mg/dL might be candidates for niacin. He says that for both men and women, an HDL of 60 mg/dL or higher is ideal.

Doctors tend to prescribe niacin as the first line of cardiovascular defense *after* patients have tried unsuccessfully to raise HDL with lifestyle changes—and there we are again with the recommendation of a healthful diet, increased and regular exercise, and of course not smoking. Also, niacin is sometimes used as an alternative treatment for patients who can't tolerate statins—for instance, because of their side effect of muscle pain. But the fact is that niacin doesn't reduce LDL anywhere near as much as statins, and LDL reduction is considered by most cardiologists to be more important than HDL increase. Still, niacin can help patients with slightly high LDL who also have low HDL and high triglycerides.

Niacin can also be used *with* statins: people who already are taking a statin to reduce LDL may be advised to take niacin to boost HDL. Dr. Nissen says the Cleveland Clinic usually waits for a few months after starting statin therapy before adding niacin, because statins slightly increase HDL—and that in turn can affect the niacin dose. The balancing act is never a simple one.

Dr. Nissen reminds patients that in therapeutic doses, niacin almost always causes flushing and side effects such as upset stomach and headache. To be on the lookout for possible liver damage, which is rare but can be serious, he recommends regular blood tests; to try to reduce the discomfort of flushing, one idea he suggests is taking niacin at bedtime, because many patients can sleep through the

The balancing act is never a simple one.

flushing. Dr. Nissen also points out that niacin users should not drink alcohol within an hour of taking niacin, because that can make flushing more intense.

Although niacin should be taken only under a doctor's supervision, it is available in over-the-counter supplements as well as by prescription. Dr. Nissen says the OTC niacin supplements may be just as effective as prescription drugs—but because supplements are more loosely regulated than medications, it is difficult to know if an OTC product has the amount of niacin listed on the label. And he warns against using any product labeled "no flush niacin," because products so labeled do not raise HDL at all.

Despite Dr. Nissen's warnings, many patients concerned about flushing and other effects of niacin do look for no-flush formulations, and some health practitioners actually recommend them. Mark A. Stengler, NMD, a naturopathic doctor and leading authority on alternative and integrated medicine, director of the La Jolla, California, Whole Health Clinic and adjunct clinical professor at the National College of Natural Medicine in Portland, Oregon, gets quite specific, saying that in his view, instead of taking aspirin, ibuprofen or naproxen regularly, patients should use an over-the-counter flush-free niacin known as *inositol hexaniacinate* or other non-flush-inducing form of niacin.

Who is right, Dr. Nissen or Dr. Stengler? Which is better, niacin or statins? As in so many other aspects of modern medicine, there unfortunately is no clear-cut answer. Health practitioners generally agree on target ranges for LDL of less than 130 mg/dL, HDL of 50 mg/dL or higher, and total cholesterol of 161 mg/dL to 199 mg/dL for healthy adults, 161 mg/dL to 180 mg/dL for people with diabetes or cardiovascular disease. Even those

numbers are not universally accepted, though, with some
doctors now arguing that total cholesterol of 160 mg/dL
or less and LDL of 70 mg/dL or less are the best targets
for people with high heart-disease risk—while those at
lower risk should aim for LDL below 100 mg/dL.

Lifestyle for Better Health

As for how to get to whatever level they recommend:
practitioners of all types generally agree that the first
thing most people should do to reduce cardiovascular
risk is to live a more-healthful lifestyle through weight
reduction, better dietary habits and regular exercise. But
there the points of agree-
Doctors tend to ment end. The main goal
prescribe a statin of cholesterol treatment is
plus niacin when to lower LDL, and statins
either drug by do this much more effec-
itself fails to have tively than niacin does. But
sufficient effect. niacin has the advantage
of raising HDL much more
than statins do and also lowering triglycerides, fats in the
blood that can increase the risk of heart disease. So niacin may be a good option for people who cannot tolerate
statins well and for those who have very low HDL and/
or high triglycerides. Niacin may also help people who
have elevated levels of small, dense LDL particles, which
increase coronary risk.

And what about the occasional practice of using
statins *plus* niacin? Doctors tend to prescribe this combination when either drug by itself fails to have sufficient effect, or when patients have low HDL and/or
high triglycerides as well as high LDL. The combination
improves cholesterol levels more than either drug alone,

but—and it seems there is always a "but" of some sort—
the question of whether the combination is better than a
statin alone for preventing heart attacks is unclear.

A major and long-awaited federal study called
into question the notion of adding niacin to statin
therapy—at least in some patients. The study, called
AIM-HIGH, involved 3,400 people with a history of
cardiovascular disease who were already taking a statin
to lower their LDL,
but still had low   *A major study found*
HDL and high   *little benefit to using*
triglycerides. Their   *niacin in patients taking*
statin doses were   *statins.*
adjusted so they
achieved an LDL target of less than 80. Some subjects
were then also given the high-dose extended-release
prescription niacin sold as Niaspan ®, with the expectation that it would offer extra protection by raising HDL
and lowering triglycerides.

However, the study was stopped early, after 32
months, when it unexpectedly became clear that the
combination group, despite its higher HDL levels, did
not have fewer heart attacks or other cardiovascular
events than the statin-only group—and actually had
slightly *more* strokes.

Now, this was a select group of older patients with
existing coronary heart disease—and the patients already
had lowered their LDL levels significantly through statin
use. Maybe something in the patient group caused the
unexpected result, and maybe things would be different
with other patients. Perhaps, once LDL is so low, raising
HDL no longer matters much—there may be little room
for further reduction in cardiac risk. So perhaps niacin,
added to statins, *can* provide added benefits for people

with a different risk profile or those who have not reduced their LDL level so dramatically.

Or maybe the results of the AIM-HIGH study
resulted from a statistical fluke. The justification for
thinking that? No previous studies on niacin found an
increased risk of stroke.

The AIM-HIGH study was certainly not the last
word—much larger studies of a niacin/statin combination continue to be done. But these studies take years
to do and additional months, at least, to interpret and
report. This is enormously frustrating for patients who,
after all, have to make decisions about their treatment
immediately, based on the most reliable available evidence at the time. It is frustrating for doctors, too, since
the only thing they can do is suggest treatment based
on the best current information—and both "best" and
"current" are slippery, ever-changing concepts.

Small wonder, then, that some health practitioners are looking for ways to avoid all the debates about
statins, niacin and other cardiovascular treatments by
seeking so-called natural alternatives to all forms of
medication.

4

The Natural Approach

I t was a brilliant slogan. "Without chemicals, life itself would be impossible." Monsanto Corporation used it in the 1960s, and it is still talked about today—both positively and negatively.

The statement happens to be true, whether or not you like the use to which Monsanto put it. Our bodies run on chemicals, depend on chemicals, manufacture chemicals all the time. No chemicals, no life. A chemical is simply a substance that has been purified and thus adapted to a specific purpose, which is what our bodies do constantly.

Our bodies run on chemicals, depend on chemicals, manufacture chemicals all the time.

Of course, what people who dislike the Monsanto slogan and its implications object to is *artificial* chemicals, ones made by a manufacturing process rather than naturally by humans, other animals or plants. These are frequently the people looking for "natural alternatives" to statins, on the basis that chemicals created by pharmaceutical companies are inferior in some way to ones created in nature.

The problem with this argument is that while some statins are indeed synthetic, some are naturally occurring compounds—the product of fermentation, which is a natural biological process. *Lovastatin*, sold under

Some statins are naturally occurring compounds. the brand names Mevacor®, Altocor® and Altoprev™, is found naturally on oyster mushrooms and red yeast rice. *Pravastatin,* sold as Pravachol®, Selektine® and Lipostat®, is a fermentation product of a bacterium called *Nocardia autotrophica.*

Simvastatin, sold as Zocor® and Lipex®, has a foot in both the natural and synthetic camps. It is fermentation-derived, but as manufactured is a synthetic derivative of a fermentation product of the bacterium *Aspergillis terreus.*

Other statins are indeed synthetic: *Atorvastatin* (Lipitor®, Torvast®); *Fluvastatin* (Lescol®); *Pitavastatin* (Livalo®, Pitava®); and *Rosuvastatin* (Crestor®).

But none of this stops people who have concerns, whether health-related or philosophical, about statin use, from insisting that there are ways to protect against heart disease without using statins—and that those ways are "more natural," however that may be defined.

The Naturopathic Prescription

Mark A. Stengler, NMD, a naturopathic doctor and leading authority on alternative and integrated medicine, founder of the Stengler Center for Integrative Medicine in Encinitas, California, is not entirely against statins. There are times when he recommends them: immediately after a heart attack to reduce inflammation, and when there is extreme elevation in total cholesterol, 400 mg/dL or higher, and/or LDL cholesterol, 200 mg/dL or higher.

At other times and for the vast majority of patients, though, Dr. Stengler says that a combination of lifestyle changes and use of supplements is better than a statin regimen. His suggestions about lifestyle are in some ways unremarkable and in line with those of medical doctors and other health practitioners: eat more-healthful foods, avoid smoking, lose weight, exercise regularly, and lower stress through practices such as deep breathing and biofeedback.

However, Dr. Stengler's suggestions stand out from those of other holistic practitioners because of their specificity, which makes them easy to understand and simple to follow for people who prefer to avoid statins.

Consume two servings a week of foods rich in omega-3 fatty acids.

Lifestyle Alternatives to Statins

- Reduce dietary saturated fat to less than 7%, and monitor saturated-fat intake by keeping a daily record, using information from food labels.

- Avoid products that contain trans fatty acids, sometimes listed as "partially hydrogenated" fats. That means staying away from deep-fried foods, commercial bakery products, packaged snack foods, most margarines, crackers, vegetable shortening and packaged cake and cookie mixes.

- Use organic olive or canola oil, or macadamia nut oil, for cooking and eating.

- Consume two servings a week of foods rich in omega-3 fatty acids, such as anchovies, Atlantic herring, sardines, tilapia and wild or canned salmon.

- Eat five to seven daily servings of fruits and vegetables.

- Consume foods containing soluble fiber, such as beans, barley, oats, peas, apples, oranges and pears.

- Eat a daily handful of nuts that are rich in monounsaturated fatty acids, such as walnuts, macadamia nuts, pistachios, almonds, hazelnuts or pecans.

- Make ground flaxseed—up to one-quarter cup daily, taken in two doses—a regular part of the day's foods by adding it to protein shakes, cereal and/or salads. Drink 10 ounces of water for every two tablespoons of flaxseed consumed, to prevent intestinal blockage.

- Consume 20 to 30 grams of soy protein daily, either in food or in protein powder.

- Reduce daily intake of simple sugars, such as those in crackers, cookies and soda, for two reasons. First, they are thought to decrease HDL or "good cholesterol." And second, lowering sugar consumption reduces the risk of elevated insulin levels, which lead to increased production of cholesterol by the liver. In these recommendations as in so many others, all bodily systems are closely interconnected.

Reduce daily intake of simple sugars, such as those in crackers, cookies and soda.

Even these dietary arrangements are not enough for everyone, Dr. Stengler says. Some people may still have elevated cholesterol levels, perhaps because of genetic factors. For them, he recommends niacin rather than statins (see Chapter 3)unless total cholesterol is above 400 mg/dL or LDL is above 200 mg/dL. Or, instead of niacin, he says patients can consider either of two other supplements: red yeast rice extract, from which lovastatin is derived, or plant sterols and stanols.

Red Yeast Rice Extract

This is what Dr. Stengler uses first, especially if high cholesterol runs in a patient's family. Red yeast rice is a fermented rice product on which red yeast, *Monascus purpureus*, has been grown. A dietary staple in China and Japan, it is commonly used by Asian-Americans in the U.S. as a natural food preservative for fish and meat. Red yeast rice extract contains an ingredient called *monacolin K*, which inhibits the action of the liver enzyme *HMG-CoA reductase*—which is involved in cholesterol synthesis.

Red yeast rice extract does have side effects.

Inhibition of cholesterol production is also essentially what statins do, but Dr. Stengler says red yeast rice extract works without creating side effects: the amount of monacolin K in red yeast rice extract is quite small compared with that in lovastatin. He believes that other ingredients in red yeast rice extract, such as additional monacolins, sterols and fatty acids, contribute to its cholesterol-lowering properties.

Red yeast rice extract is taken in capsule form; Dr. Stengler uses it for people with total cholesterol of 200 mg/dL to 240 mg/dL; LDL of 150 mg/dL to 190 mg/dL; and/or triglycerides of 160 mg/dL to 200 mg/dL. He says it can reduce total cholesterol by 11% to 32%, LDL by up to 22%, and triglycerides by 12% to 19%.

Red yeast rice extract is not without side effects. It may cause mild heartburn, dizziness and gas for a few days to a week. People who have an existing liver disorder, particularly hepatitis, should not use red yeast rice extract, because it may stress the liver. And pregnant or breast-feeding women should avoid red yeast rice extract, since its safety has not been studied in those groups. Dr. Stengler recommends taking 50 mg to 100 mg of coenzyme Q10 (CoQ10) daily when using red yeast rice extract, because the extract may deplete the body's supply of this naturally occurring substance—which helps produce energy in cells.

Plant Sterols and Stanols

For people whose cholesterol picture does not improve with red yeast rice extract after eight to 12 weeks—as measured by a blood test comparing cholesterol levels with what they were before starting to use the extract—Dr. Stengler recommends switching to plant sterols, which are components of plant-cell membranes that resemble cholesterol in animals; and plant stanols, which are derived from sterols. Since 2000, the Food and Drug Administration has allowed the use of product labels that make health claims related to plant sterol esters and stanol esters—substances that holistic practitioners have advocated for many years as ways to reduce cardiovascular risks.

Plant sterols and stanols are present in small quantities in many fruits, vegetables, nuts, seeds, cereals, legumes, vegetable oils and other plant sources. There are a few foods that have them added, including certain salad dressings and snack bars, and spreads such as Benecol and Promise. Dr. Stengler says that someone

who uses one to two tablespoons of margarine daily
and switches to a spread with stanols may reduce LDL
levels by up to 10%. But for maximum effectiveness, he
suggests supplementation, not just replacement: a daily
supplement that contains two to three grams of plant
sterols—or the specific sterol known as beta-sitosterol—
in divided doses with food.

Like red yeast rice extract, plant sterols and stanols
do have side effects, although the FDA deems them
"generally recognized as safe." There is research indicating that the body's levels of beta-carotene, a precursor
of vitamin A, fall slightly in people who take sterols
or stanols. Therefore, Dr. Stengler recommends that
people using these plant substances take a multivitamin
containing beta-carotene daily and also eat foods with
high concentrations of beta-carotene, such as carrots,
melons and tomatoes.

Taking a Wider View

It is worth spending a fairly extensive amount of time
on Dr. Stengler's approach and recommendations,
because they represent one form of thinking about cardiovascular disease and the role of statins in preventing
it. Few of Dr. Stengler's recommendations are outside
the standard realm of what holistic practitioners argue
for, but he makes his suggestions with more specificity
and greater attention to traditional medical alternatives than do practitioners who have a visceral dislike
of pharmaceutical companies' products and of "non-
natural" treatment in general.

A pragmatist, Dr. Stengler does recommend use
of statins in certain circumstances, but he argues that
for most people, they are simply not necessary and

have the potential to do more harm than good. The lifestyle modifications and supplementation that he recommends have fewer side effects, he believes, and are better for the body's overall health than "popping a pill" and expecting it to do the heavy lifting of cardiac-disease protection.

Few medical doctors would disagree with part of this—indeed, a large part. Doctors routinely urge overweight patients to lose weight, sedentary ones to move around and exercise more, smokers to quit, people who consume large amounts of red meat to reduce their consumption and focus more on poultry and fish, and patients who eat little produce to increase their intake of fruits and vegetables. And there is a big advantage to lifestyle changes over medication use: they are self-sustaining *as long as patients adopt them and maintain them*. In other words, to the extent that patients live in a more-healthful way, they will improve their health—by definition. The compliance issue disappears: everyday life *is* the compliance. But the cardiac consequences of weight gain, lack of exercise and suboptimal diet generally do not appear until well into a person's adult life, by which time the habits of decades are extremely difficult to break.

Medical and naturopathic doctors agree on many recommendations.

Although a new habit can theoretically become routine in about a month, this is unrealistic when it comes to the most basic elements of everyday life, which certainly include food and mobility. Close supervision of lifestyle-changing attempts is crucial until the changes take hold, but this sort of supervision is very difficult for medical doctors to provide: it is not their primary treatment approach, which is oriented toward identifying and curing illness, and it is strongly discouraged by the government and insurance industry, whose reimbursement protocols put a premium on short patient visits—and as few of them as possible for each complaint.

On the other hand, patients who choose to see holistic practitioners are doing so because they want what is usually called an "alternative" approach to health, and the practitioners themselves tend to build their practices around a focus on the whole patient rather than his or her collection of symptoms.

Therefore, people predisposed to see holistic practitioners may be more willing to make the lifestyle changes that those practitioners urge, and the practitioners may be more willing to monitor and encourage them as they do so.

People who see holistic practitioners may be more willing to make the lifestyle changes that those practitioners urge.

This becomes a self-reinforcing system that can indeed be of considerable value to some people and obviate the necessity of their taking medication for the rest of their lives.

Differing Treatment Models

But that applies to some people, not all, and indeed not the majority. For a wide variety of societal and sociopolitical reasons, most people continue to turn to medical doctors for health care, which is why holistic practitioners are considered to be part of "alternative medicine." Primary medical care still uses the diagnose-and-cure model, which works very well for acute illness but less well for chronic conditions, such as the decades-long cardiovascular issues than eventually kill more Americans than does any other cause.

Furthermore, the vast majority of patients are simply not sufficiently motivated to make significant lifestyle changes that require them to eat differently, move differently, schedule their time differently—in short, to approach their lives differently. It is useless to argue that more people *should* make those changes, although in fact many patients will acknowledge that they should, for example, exercise daily, but just don't have the time, or are too tired, or work too many hours, or have too many stresses at home, or some combination of those or other factors. It would require considerable counseling time—which medical doctors are neither trained nor inclined to provide, and which psychologists and psychiatrists are generally not reimbursed for providing—to reorient most patients' thinking sufficiently to get them to make the sorts of changes in their busy, time-pressed lives that they ideally "should" make.

Statin use and complementary approaches are not mutually exclusive.

Therefore, as admirable as alternative and holistic approaches to cardiovascular health may be, and as effective as they may be for some people, they are unlikely to become the dominant method of cholesterol control in light of the availability of statins.

It is worth pointing out that the statin and complementary approaches are not mutually exclusive. Brent A. Bauer, MD, director of the Complementary and Integrative Medicine Program and a physician in the department of internal medicine at the Mayo Clinic in Rochester, Minnesota, as well as a professor of medicine at the Mayo Medical School, points out that people with higher cholesterol levels can combine a butter substitute such as Benecol or Promise with a statin drug and obtain better cholesterol improvement than with either approach alone. For example, he says, people who eat the equivalent of three pats of one of these butter substitutes daily can achieve reductions of 10% to 20% in LDL—in addition to the reductions achieved with medications.

And just as significantly, Dr. Bauer points out that in some cases of taking a combined approach to cholesterol control, the statin dose can be reduced—lowering the risk of side effects.

This issue of side effects emerges again and again when it comes to statins and is one of the central elements of the statin dilemma. Because side effects are so central to arguments for and against statins, it is important to examine them in detail, in terms of both their likelihood and their severity.

The issue of side effects emerges again and again when it comes to statins.

5

Worst-Case Planning

Baycol® worked. The most notorious of all statins did what it was supposed to do: it lowered cholesterol effectively. Bearing the chemical name *cerivastatin* and also sold as Lipobay®, the synthetic statin was manufactured and sold by Germany-based Bayer A.G. in the late 1990s. The U.S. Food and Drug Administration approved it in 1997.

The problem was that Baycol® also did things it was *not* supposed to do and was taken off the market in August 2001.

World Health Organization (WHO) Alert

Bayer Pharmaceutical Division has announced its decision to withdraw Baycol (cerivastatin) from the U.S. market following reports of rhabdomyolysis, a severe muscle adverse reaction that can sometimes have fatal consequences. The FDA has agreed with and supported this decision.

Baycol (cerivastatin) was initially approved in the U.S. in 1997. It belongs to a group of cholesterol lowering drugs referred to as "statins." While all statins could potentially cause this dangerous muscle reaction, rhabdomyolysis appears more frequent with cerivastatin, especially when used in high doses, in the elderly, or when taken along with gemfibrozil, another cholesterol lowering drug. In this connection it may be noted that Bayer has withdrawn all dosages of Baycol / Lipobay with immediate effect throughout the world (except in Japan where gemfibrozil is not available). The company is also withdrawing current market supplies of the product.

Lovastatin (Mevacor), pravastatin (Pravachol), simvastatin (Zocor), fluvastatin (Lescol) and atorvastatin (Lipitor) are five other statins that may be used as alternatives to cerivastatin.

Cerivastatin

The WHO statement is notable on several levels, both for what it says and for what it omits. This was a voluntary recall, not one mandated by the FDA, although the FDA "agreed with and supported" Bayer's decision. Baycol®, the statement notes, is not the only statin that can cause rhabdomyolysis: "all statins could potentially cause this dangerous muscle reaction." The dangerous side effect is most common when Baycol® is "used in high doses" or "along with gemfibrozil, another cholesterol lowering drug." Therefore, Bayer planned to continue selling Baycol® in Japan, "where gemfibrozil is not available."

What Was Unsaid

As for what the statement does not say: Baycol® was at the time available in Japan only in lower doses; this was another factor in Bayer's decision to keep selling the statin there. That decision was later reversed, and Baycol® was withdrawn worldwide within a few weeks of the WHO announcement. Bayer informed patients and the German government of the withdrawal of Baycol® only after letting financial markets know what was going on—timing that earned the company a strong rebuke from German Health Minister Ulla Schmidt Bayer, who has no relation to the company.

The company was caught in a legal bind, as it pointed out, insisting that it acted to withdraw the drug and informed doctors and pharmacists as early as possible, subject to its legal obligation to inform financial markets immediately of any developments that could affect the company's share price. Indeed, Bayer's stock price fell 25% within weeks of the withdrawal of Baycol®.

Without getting into the political and legal ramifications of Bayer's decision, and the company's relationship with the German government—subsequent lawsuits involving Baycol® enriched many lawyers worldwide—the fact is that, medically, Bayer's decision to pull Baycol® from the market was made based on information that the company could not have known at the time the drug was approved for use. The clinical trials on the basis of which drugs are approved for

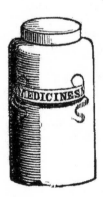

widespread patient use are, by definition, *trials*, using a limited number of people to try to indicate what will probably happen when the medication is available to a much larger group of patients in the real world. People with severe diseases and various complicating health factors are systematically excluded from the trials, yet it is these very people, often older and/or sicker than those participating in trials, who are most likely to be vulnerable to medications' side effects.

Thus, the incidence of side effects, even dangerous ones, may be too small in a trial to become cause for alarm; but when a drug is taken by thousands, hundreds of thousands or millions of people, severe side effects may become far more apparent and worrisome. This is why the FDA and other government agencies that oversee medication use require companies to keep monitoring their drugs after approval. All companies do this for all their medicines.

Deaths from Baycol®

What happened with Baycol® was that 52 people died, mostly from the rapid destruction of skeletal muscle known as rhabdomyolysis—and the kidney failure that rhabdomyolysis can cause. This is not a huge number in absolute or percentage terms, and the same condition is known to occur with other statins—but the incidence of rhabdomyolysis was 16 to 80 times as high with Baycol® as with other statins. That was more than enough reason to withdraw the drug.

In the inevitable lawsuits after the withdrawal, company documents were released that revealed that muscle weakness, myopathy, was also a side effect of Baycol®, especially when the drug was taken in larger doses. But other statins have this same dose-dependent side effect, and this by itself would probably not have led Bayer to withdraw the medicine. The rhabdomyolysis incidence, though, was an extremely serious matter.

The body has three types of muscle: smooth muscle, heart muscle and skeletal muscle. It is skeletal muscle, which moves the skeleton at the joints, that is affected by rhabdomyolysis. The condition has many causes. It is most often seen in patients who have suffered muscle trauma, crush injuries, severe burns, child abuse or physical torture. Prolonged coma can cause it; so can extended lying on the ground—for instance, being unconscious for several hours. Serious seizures can result in rhabdomyolysis; so can extreme physical activity, such as running a marathon. Viruses, bacteria, some inflammatory diseases, even some bites from venomous snakes can cause it. And statins are not the only medicines with rhabdomyolysis as a side effect—some Parkinson's disease medications, psychiatric medicines, HIV treatments, and even the gout treatment colchicine can cause it.

It is skeletal muscle that is affected by rhabdomyolysis.

What happens in rhabdomyolysis is that skeletal muscle is rapidly destroyed, resulting in leakage of the muscle protein *myoglobin* into the urine. Symptoms may include muscle aches and pain, stiffness, muscle weakness, and darkening of urine to a red or even cola color. Sometimes, rhabdomyolysis has no significant symptoms. In serious cases, though, its complications can be severe and even fatal. For example, it may cause abnormality of electrolytes in the blood: the release into the bloodstream of the contents of damaged muscle cells can lead to high levels of potassium, a condition known as *hyperkalemia*, and phosphorus, *hyperphosphatemia*. The greatest danger, though, is kidney failure: the filtration tubes of the kidneys can be blocked by muscle proteins, reducing and eventually fatally impairing kidney function.

This is what happened to dozens of users of Baycol®. The exact reasons for the high incidence of rhabdomyolysis in Baycol® users are unknown and will likely nev-

er be known—it is not as if anyone is going to run clinical trials using a medicine withdrawn from the market
because of the dangers it poses. In fact, for a time, the
extent of the danger was unclear. Doctors discovered
that risks were higher in patients using *fibrates* as cardiovascular drugs supplementing the statin—mainly a
medicine called Lopid, chemical name *gemfibrozil*. Risks
also increased in patients
using the highest dose of *The exact reasons*
Baycol®: 0.8 mg/day. Bayer *for the effects of*
actually added a warning *Baycol® will likely*
against use of both Baycol® *never be known.*
and gemfibrozil to the Bay-
col® package 18 months after the drug interaction was
found. But as evidence mounted of the greater dangers
of Baycol®, compared with other statins, the manufacturer decided to take the drug off the market.

A Much Higher Incidence

In addition to the 52 deaths associated with Baycol®,
385 non-fatal cases of rhabdomyolysis were reported.
This meant that, taken as a whole, the incidence of
rhabdomyolysis with Baycol® was five to 10 times as
high as its incidence with other statins. In statistical
terms, the complication remained rare, but that was
small comfort to affected patients and families—and
in light of the availability of other statins with less-
frequent, less-onerous side effects, the withdrawal of
Baycol® made perfect sense and was in fact necessary.

Rhabdomyolysis is the most serious muscular side
effect of statin use, but it is certainly not the only one,
and not the most common. There are many kinds of
myopathy, a word that simply means "muscle disease,"

associated with statins. In fact, one of the warnings given out to patients taking these medications is that they may be at risk for muscle pain or even rhabdomyolysis, which patients are usually told means "muscle breakdown." Doctors usually recommend to patients that if they have muscle pain while taking a statin, especially at a high dose, they seek immediate medical help—although, in fact, emergency-room visits are usually useless for a complaint as vague as painful muscles.

The frequency of statin-associated myopathy is a subject of debate and is part of the controversy over statins, with those opposed to them saying myopathy is more common than generally believed and those favoring them, including manufacturers, saying myopathy is uncommon, generally mild, and usually a minor tradeoff for the benefits that statins provide.

In an attempt to find out just how common statin-induced myopathy is, researchers at the University of Washington looked at computerized pharmacy data to review the electronic medical records of statin users. Importantly, they did not rely on the specific medical diagnostic code for statin-related rhabdomyolysis to track down the number of cases, since myopathy may not be serious enough to be called rhabdomyolysis and since doctors have some discretion about how they code patient illnesses. For the same reason, the researchers did not rely on billing data coded to rhabdomyolysis.

The frequency of statin-associated myopathy is a subject of debate and is part of the controversy over statins.

The researchers came up with 292 statin users who were coded for muscle breakdown, but only 22 cases of statin-related muscle injury. In addition, they found seven cases of statin-related myopathy using other methods, for a total of 29 cases; 26 of those required hospitalization. There were no deaths.

Misleading Diagnostic Codes

The University of Washington study confirmed the FDA warning about use of high-dose statins, which, it is generally agreed, increase the risk of myopathy. And the study showed—although this was not its purpose—that tracking down complications using diagnostic codes can be misleading, and can lead to overestimating the incidence of those side effects—292 codes for muscle breakdown were found, but only 29 turned out to be statin-related. The most reasonable and conservative conclusion would seem to be that actual muscle breakdown associated with statins—that is, rhabdomyolysis—is very rare, but vague muscle aches are more common.

It is important to remember that side effects occur with *all* medicines. Aspirin can cause gastric upset and bleeding; pain relievers containing codeine, such as Tylenol® 2 and Tylenol® 3, can cause mental fuzziness and disorientation; even a mild blood-pressure drug, such as lisinopril, may cause chest pain, stomach pain and fatigue. Systemic medicines affect the entire bodily system—a fact that doctors often neglect to mention and patients tend to ignore. *Significant* side effects of statins, such as rhabdomyolysis, are rare, but lesser ones are more common. So the question is: do the side effects significantly change the risk-benefit ratio of the drugs? The answer may depend on why you are taking—or considering taking—statins and what your existing cardiac profile is.

Statin Chemical Names and Brand Names

Atorvastatin: Lipitor®

Fluvastatin: Lescol®

Lovastatin: Mevacor® or Altoprev™

Pravastatin: Pravachol®

Rosuvastatin calcium: Crestor®

Simvastatin: Zocor®

Statin Combination Medicines

Atorvastatin + amlodipine: Caduet®

Lovastatin + niacin: Advicor®

Simvastatin + ezetimibe: Vytorin™

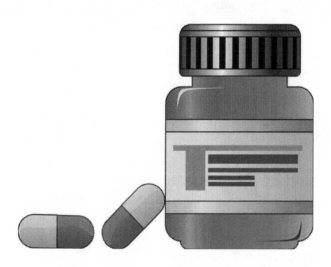

6

The Primary-Prevention Controversy

Much of the medical argument about statins turns on their use in primary prevention of cardiovascular disease—that is, prescribing them to patients who have risk factors for heart trouble but have not actually had a heart attack. A lot of the argument turns on the definition of the word "healthy" and the phrase "otherwise healthy."

Doctors who believe that someone is healthy or otherwise healthy despite elevated cholesterol levels and a less-than-optimal balance of HDL and LDL tend to bristle at the idea of medicating these individuals with powerful drugs that have known and potentially serious side effects. Doctors who believe that people with elevated lipid levels are *seemingly* healthy—are, in effect, cardiovascular events waiting to happen—tend to feel that statins' undoubted benefits outweigh their risks.

Doctors on both sides of this issue agree that good diet and exercise are the foundations of heart health, but they tend to disagree on whether that is enough. Those favoring statins point out that even people who eat well and exercise regularly may have known risk factors for cardiac events, and that such risk factors can be mitigated by statins. Those opposing statins tend to say that patients adhering to a healthful lifestyle are otherwise healthy even if some of their blood markers are suboptimal—and that such patients should not be put on potent medicines for the rest of their lives just because of their blood-test results.

Roger S. Blumenthal, MD, professor of medicine and director of the Johns Hopkins Ciccarone Center for the Prevention of Heart Disease in Baltimore, is a strong advocate of primary-prevention statin therapy. Diet and exercise are simply not enough to prevent heart attack in many people, he says, and in fact elevated levels of LDL are a significant predictor of heart trouble to come—so giving statins to patients with high LDL means protecting them; they are not really healthy in cardiovascular terms, but are more like

Doctors on both sides of the statin issue agree that good diet and exercise are the foundations of heart health.

accidents waiting to happen. Dr. Blumenthal points out that trials have shown reductions in cardiovascular events of 30% to 40% with the use of a statin.

The problem with heart disease, Dr. Blumenthal argues, is that it takes decades to manifest. The first time it shows up may be with a heart attack or stroke—at which point prescribing a statin, while certainly possible, is less than optimal. Not everyone should get statins, Dr. Blumenthal says, but those shown to be at high risk for heart disease should.

Dr. Blumenthal believes that many claims about statins' side effects are exaggerated or anecdotal—a more strongly argued position than those of many other pro-statin physicians. Even to the extent that side effects do occur, he believes the drugs can prolong life while reducing patient suffering from heart attacks, strokes and bypass surgery. And he adds that he does not accept a common argument among statin opponents, that lifestyle changes are cheaper than drugs—because generic statins such as simvastatin and atorvastatin cost only about $50 a year, which is much less than the cost of a year's worth of fruits and vegetables. A combination of improved lifestyle with statin use is, he argues, the best approach.

Rita Redberg, MD, a professor of medicine and director of women's cardiovascular services at the University of California, San Francisco, does not buy Dr. Blumenthal's arguments. In a point-counterpoint presentation in *The Wall Street Journal*, she said that statins do *not* prevent heart disease, extend life or improve quality of

Simvastatin

life—and should not be used in people with elevated cholesterol who are otherwise healthy. The side effects of statins and the lack of long-term proof that statin users live longer than non-users mean the drugs are over-prescribed, without adequate evidence for their use. Dr. Redberg argues that statins undeniably—not anecdotally—harm some people by increasing their risk for developing diabetes and by causing memory loss, muscle weakness, stomach distress, and various aches and pains.

Diet Plus Exercise

Diet and exercise alone are enough for people who have not yet had cardiac events, Dr. Redberg argues. She told the *Journal* that if we as a nation were to spend a small fraction of the annual cost of statins on making fruits and vegetables and physical activity more accessible, the effect on heart disease would be far greater than anything statins can do—and there

> *Efforts toward better lifestyles "should start in the school system."*
>
> —Rita Redberg, M.D.

would also be positive effects on high blood pressure, diabetes, cancer and overall life span. However, she downplayed the major societal changes that her prescription would entail, acknowledging that her approach requires commitment on many levels, from physicians to public-health officials, but saying that she considers it "entirely feasible."

Given the dysfunctional politics in the United States, that is at best an arguable statement. For example, Dr. Redberg suggests that efforts toward better lifestyles should start in the school system, where there could be more physical education and greater improvement in the nutritional value of school lunches and snacks.

Some of this is in fact going on, but attempts to change the composition of school lunches to make them more healthful have also had unintended consequences, including students falling asleep in afternoon classes

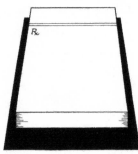

and protests by the students themselves. Also, there is
no evidence that mandated additional physical activity
improves students' body-mass-index measurements—
that is, their BMI numbers—because the time spent
on such activity is taken from some other activity that
frequently generates just about the same amount of
physical benefit.

Dr. Redberg's objections to statins come down to
two: first, that it may be true that lifestyle improvements alone cannot lower cholesterol, but that lower
cholesterol does not necessarily translate into increased
lifespan or other improved clinical outcomes—in other
words, that
people with *"The initiation of medication*
elevated cho- *motivates patients because*
lesterol may be *they better realize how*
just as healthy, *serious their cardiovascular*
overall, as ones *risk actually is."*
with lower lev-
els; and, second, that statins are "a moral hazard." She
believes that some people will make less effort to follow
a healthful diet and get regular exercise "because they
feel falsely reassured by their medications."

This latter assertion gets statin supporters such as
Dr. Blumenthal up in arms. Most of his patients are by
no means falsely reassured by their medications, he told
the *Journal.* Quite the opposite: he said taking statins
motivates people, because it makes them better realize
how serious their cardiovascular risk actually is. "If your
doctor recommended a statin to you because of high
risk of heart disease," Dr. Blumenthal asked, "would you
eat more hamburgers because of this safety net or would
you try to exercise a little more?"

Taking out the moral part of the equation—which is arguable in whatever way doctors and patients choose to argue it—there remain differing interpretations of statin studies on the issue of primary prevention. Dr. Blumenthal points to the West of Scotland Prevention Study of 6,600 Scottish men who had not had heart attacks and who showed a decrease in mortality rates after five years with statin therapy. Dr. Redberg addresses the same study, saying it was flawed because it looked at a high-risk group for whom the benefits of statins were most likely to outweigh the risks: all subjects were men, 80% were current or former smokers and had body mass index (BMI) in the overweight or obese range, and some had heart disease.

> *"Would you eat more hamburgers because of this safety net or would you try to exercise a little more?"*
> —Roger S. Blumenthal, M.D.

The Wall Street Journal may seem an unlikely place for a debate of this type, but there is plenty of the same sort of thing in medical publications. In fact, Dr. Redberg coauthored an editorial in *Archives of Internal Medicine* that said, in part, that using statins for people without coronary artery disease is a clear example of the widespread use of medications with known negative effects—without data showing patient benefit.

Subsequently, Dr. Blumenthal was one of seven physicians signing a research letter in the same journal stating that "there is compelling evidence to support the use of statins for primary prevention in patients at high risk" of developing heart disease within the next decade. Dr. Blumenthal and his fellow authors agreed that statins are unlikely to be helpful to low-cardiac-risk patients, but they said that the distinction between low-risk and high-risk is crucial. For example, patients not known to have coronary heart disease—but who do have such conditions as diabetes, hypertension, hyperlipidemia, and tobacco use—have an increased risk of heart trouble and therefore are likely to benefit from using statins for primary prevention.

How can a patient make sense of all this? Unfortunately, the answer is: not very easily. When experts come to different conclusions from the same data, a patient's reaction may range from "a plague on both your houses" to simple acceptance of whatever the patient's doctor happens to recommend—patients with pro-statin doctors take statins while ones with anti-statin doctors do not. This is poor decision-making, although certainly understandable: if there is no consensus among doctors, how can patients possibly make the right decision?

One Area of Agreement

Actually, there is a consensus—Dr. Blumenthal says that the carefully considered use of cholesterol-lowering medicines is recommended in clinical guidelines not only in the United States but also in Canada and Europe. He adds that "it's sort of silly to have this conversation" about not giving cholesterol-lowering medicines to people with risk factors for coronary heart disease. In fact, he says that the "extreme point

If there is no consensus among doctors, how can patients possibly make the right decision?

of view" of statin opponents "would be considered malpractice" in most or all U.S. states. However, statin opponents hold their viewpoint intensely, even passion-ately, and argue that for certain patient populations—women, for example—there is even less evidence of statins' benefits than for others.

Much of the argument turns on drawing the line about *selective* use of statins—and also on philosophy. Some doctors say the possession of cardiac risk factors provides sufficient information on drawing the line on statin use; others say it does not—and those with this viewpoint tend to have strong feelings about how pa-tients should behave, should eat, and should live their everyday lives. Doctors actually agree about lifestyle issues on both sides of the primary-prevention debate, but those favoring statins for primary prevention tend to be less sanguine than statin opponents about actu-ally getting people to make lifestyle changes—in many cases, very significant ones. When it comes to second-ary prevention, however, the viewpoints come together much more clearly.

7

After a Heart Attack

L et us go back for a moment to the early days of statins. They were first introduced in 1987 as a way to lower blood cholesterol levels by affecting how much of the substance the liver produces, how much the intestines absorb, or how much circulates in the bloodstream. Pioneering Japanese microbiologist Akira Endo is the discoverer of the first statin, but scarcely the only researcher to have made important discoveries about them. For example, research into statins—specifically for findings relating to how cholesterol metabolism is regulated—won the 1985 Nobel Prize in Physiology or Medicine for Michael Brown, MD, and Joseph Goldstein, MD.

And even Akira Endo was not the first explorer in this field. During the Korean War, researchers were shocked to learn from autopsy studies that 75% of soldiers killed in Korea—whose average age was only 22—were already showing signs of coronary plaque buildup. At the same time, scientists were studying laboratory animals, feeding them a then-typical American diet of steak, mashed potatoes and gravy, mixed with banana as a flavor enhancer so the animals, rhesus monkeys, would eat it. After a short time, the monkeys went from having healthy arteries to having severe atherosclerosis. Years later, in the 1970s, scientists discovered that by changing the monkeys' diet back to bananas and greens, the damage to the animals' arteries could be reversed. This set the stage for arguments in favor of dietary modification as defense against heart disease—and also paved the way for the intensive search for a cholesterol-lowering medication.

The Approval Process

But why were statins approved in the first place? This is not a trivial question, and its answer is not an obvious one. Medications are granted approval for specific applications; once they gain that approval, pharmaceutical manufacturers immediately look for ways to get it expanded so the newly available medicine can be used by more people and generate more sales. There is nothing sinister about this: developing a new drug takes many years and costs hundreds of millions of dollars, so it is reasonable for

Developing a new drug takes many years and costs hundreds of millions of dollars.

a manufacturer to want to sell as much of the medicine as possible during the patent-protection period, before generic versions of the drug can be made. And clinical trials are expensive and time-consuming—running them for all possible uses of a drug prior to requesting approval to sell the medicine would be prohibitively costly, would significantly delay introduction of the medicine, and could lead to the needless deaths of many people whose lives could have been saved if the drug had been available sooner.

Nevertheless, the system has weaknesses and is subject to abuse. It encourages pharmaceutical firms to get drugs to market quickly, because the 20-year U.S. patent protection is backdated to the patent application, which normally is submitted before clinical trials begin; therefore, the longer the trials last, the less time a company has to market its new drug exclusively—the exclusivity period can be as little as seven years. Also, the system leads some doctors to prescribe medicines on an off-label basis, meaning to have them used for purposes other than the approved ones or by people for whom the drugs were not okayed—a medicine accepted as safe for people up to age 49, for example, may be used on people over age 60. The system also encourages manufacturers to promote the possibility of drug use for purposes far from those originally intended—statins, it has been suggested, may be helpful in treating every-thing from Alzheimer's disease and multiple sclerosis to swine flu; and there is some evidence that this may be so, but other evidence that it is not.

Why Statins Were Approved

The one use for which approved drugs can be counted on to work as expected is the use for which they were granted approval in the first place. And for statins, that approval was for use *after a heart attack*. The notion that statins could also be useful to prevent a heart attack in the first place, while a logical extension of the original approval and one on which many—but not all—doc-tors agree, was not in the original approval.

This matters to patients who have had heart attacks and to their families, because with all the controversy about statins, their basic efficacy for the purpose for which they were originally approved has never been seri-ously doubted. *Statins save the lives of heart-attack victims.* The Scandinavian Simvastatin Survival Study, which is still considered definitive although it dates to 1994, showed that treating patients with pre-existing heart disease decreased their chance of dying within five years

from 12% without statins to 8% with them. That is a
drop of one-third, or 33%—a really significant decrease.

Furthermore, the study found that heart patients'
five-year likelihood of cardiac death, heart attack, or
needing heart surgery fell from about 30% without
statins to around 20% with them—again, a drop of
one-third, or 33%.

Statins are largely responsible for cutting Americans' death rate from heart disease by 50%, which is an
extraordinary amount, between 1980 and 2000—an amaz-
ingly short time period for so precipitous a drop. Centers
for Disease Control and Prevention statistics show that
the rate was 543 deaths per 100,000 men in 1980 and
269 per 100,000 in 2000. For women, the rate was 263
per 100,000 in 1980 and 134
Statins save the   per 100,000 in 2000. Based on
lives of heart-   the U.S. population in 2000,
attack victims.   that changed rate means that
340,000 fewer Americans died
of heart disease than would have died from it 20 years
earlier. It is an understatement to call that a remarkable
improvement, even more so because Americans' diets did
not become more healthful during this time—despite the
urging of health-care professionals, politicians and others—and the percentage of overweight and obese people
in the United States, which means people at greater risk of
heart attack, grew inexorably.

The Debate Continues

Nevertheless, statins are not solely responsible for
these very impressive numbers, and the extent to which
their use for primary prevention has anything to do
with the decline in cardiac deaths remains much debat-
ed. One other factor, for example, could be improved

diagnostic tools that made it easy to detect heart
disease earlier and treat it more aggressively—although
it is worth pointing out that such treatment would
itself almost always have
involved statins beginning   *Early, aggressive*
in the late 1980s. In any   *statin use after a*
case, there is no question   *heart attack sig-*
that statins have been a   *nificantly reduced*
significant contributing   *patients' long-term*
factor to the great decline   *incidence of another*
in cardiac death, even if   *heart attack.*
how significant is unquan-
tifiable. "There's no doubt that the discovery of statins
has saved countless lives," says Glenn Braunstein, MD,
professor and chairman of the Department of Medicine
at Cedars-Sinai Medical Center in Los Angeles and
holder of the James R. Klinenberg Chair in Medicine.

There is now very little argument about the efficacy of
giving statins quickly after a heart attack to reduce the risk
of another one. This was not always clear: for years, physicians traditionally took a moderate approach to lowering
cholesterol in their heart patients after the patients' discharge from the hospital, typically trying to reduce cholesterol levels by beginning with dietary approaches and then
slowly adding or increasing the use of statins.

But as far back as the early 2000s, this treatment
model was starting to be found wanting. In 2004,
cardiologists Michael Blazing, MD, of Duke Clinical
Research Institute in North Carolina, and James de
Lemos, MD, from the University of Texas Southwest-
ern Medical Center in Dallas, working with a team
of investigators from their centers and Brigham and
Women's Hospital in Boston, found that early, aggressive statin use after a heart attack significantly reduced
patients' long-term incidence of another heart attack,

death from heart attack, stroke, or readmission to the hospital for a cardiac event. This study followed ones that had shown the benefits of statins in reducing the risk of heart attack in patients with stable coronary artery disease or those at risk for a future heart attack. By the time the Blazing/de Lemos study was presented to the European Society of Cardiology, the frequency of doctors giving patients statins in the hospital shortly after treatment for their heart-attack symptoms was rising significantly.

And this was not the first research to show benefits from this protocol. A Swedish study published in *Journal of the American Medical Association* in 2001 found that heart-attack patients with elevated cholesterol

> *"There's no doubt that the discovery of statins has saved countless lives."*
> —Glenn Braunstein, M.D.

levels who were placed on statins prior to their hospital discharge experienced a 25% reduction in mortality over the next 12 months, compared to similar patients not treated with statins. And even that study built on earlier data supporting the prompt use of statins after heart attacks.

So: statins reduce cholesterol. They protect people who have had a heart attack against having a second one. They do exactly what researchers dating back to the days of the Korean War hoped: reverse the effects on cardiac health of arteries that have become clogged. There is no doubt that if you have a heart attack, you want to be on statins while still in the hospital—and continue on them for the rest of your life.

But what if you were *already* on statins and had a heart attack anyway? A study published in *European Heart Journal* dealt with this very subject. The study was done by Stella S. Daskalopoulou, MD, and colleagues from McGill University and the University of Washington. It followed up people in the United Kingdom who had survived a myocardial infarction—heart attack—between January 1, 2002 and December 31, 2004. These were people who had survived at least 90 days after their first heart attack, were at least 20 years old, and had a minimum of three consecutive years of records in the General Practice Research Database or GPRD, which collects information on the health of more than three million people through 400 GP practices across the United Kingdom.

Differences in Use

The researchers divided these people into four groups, depending on their statin use around the time of their heart attack. These groups were: those who did not use statins 90 days before or after their heart attack; those who used statins before and after their heart attack; those who did not use statins before their heart attack but used them afterwards; and those who used statins before their heart attack but did not use them afterwards.

Then the researchers compared the survival of the four groups, looking at all causes of mortality, between 90 days and one year after the heart attack. This let them look at the effects that different patterns of statin use around the time of a heart attack had on survival. They also took into account other factors that might have had an effect, such as age, sex, smoking, alcohol use, obesity, and number of hospitalizations.

In all, 9,939 survivors were included in this study. Of those, 2,124 had not used statins for 90 days before or after the event; 137 had been taking statins before but did not take them afterwards; 5,652 did not take statins before their event but took them afterwards; and 2,026 were taking statins both before and after.

Compared to people who never took statins, those who started taking them after their heart attack were less likely to die after one year, while those who stopped using statins after their heart attack were at increased risk of dying after one year. Those who took statins both before and after their event were not statistically different from those who never took statins.

The number of patients who stopped taking statins after their heart attack was small, but the conclusion seems clear: there is a seriously harmful effect of stopping statins—those people who did not continue to take them after their heart attack were 88% more likely to die during the one-year followup. So yes, statins may fail to prevent a first heart attack—even proponents of using them for primary prevention

Patients who stopped using statins after their heart attack were at increased risk of dying after one year.

accept this. But if they do fail, patients should continue taking them anyway: their cholesterol-lowering ability is important in preventing further, possibly fatal cardiac consequences.

But why? That is actually a good question, and a reason for the continuing controversy about who should use statins and for what purpose. How exactly do cholesterol levels predict vulnerability to heart attack?

You might think the answer is obvious, since the notion that high cholesterol is bad and is a major cardiac risk factor is now so widely accepted. But no—the situation is not as straightforward as most people believe.

Total Cholesterol and Heart Health

Now, many people know that the total amount of cholesterol in the body is not by itself a determinant of heart health. This is where the discussion of lipids— HDL, LDL and the other types—comes in. Levels of HDL, so-called "good cholesterol," and LDL, so-called "bad cholesterol," matter, as do triglyceride levels; the ratio of triglycerides to HDL; and the ratio of total cholesterol to HDL.

Then, to make matters even more confusing—and make no mistake, they *are* confusing—there are different sizes of cholesterol particles: small and large particles of LDL, HDL, and triglycerides. And they have different effects. Small, dense particles are dangerous, because they can easily penetrate arteries; large, fluffy particles tend to bounce off artery walls without doing damage, so having a lot of them is not dangerous, even if total cholesterol is high.

The *type* of cholesterol matters, too: oxidized or not. The primary danger from cholesterol relates to small, dense, oxidized LDL particles that start building up plaque or cholesterol deposits in arteries.

Where do statins fit into all this? They lower LDL, and that can be a good thing—but they do not lower selectively, by targeting the dangerous oxidized form, nor do they significantly raise HDL to improve the various ratios that are important for cardiac health. And—just to make matters even more complicated— there are now questions as to whether *raising* HDL makes a difference in health, even though *measuring* it does appear helpful as a guide to cardiac risk. This is counterintuitive, but it is the direction in which recent research points. Robert Eckel, MD, past president of the

8

The Cholesterol Quandary

There is a reason for the old joke about why doctors "practice" medicine: they have to keep at
it until they can get it right. The reason is that
new medical information constantly becomes available, and even the interpretation of currently available
information is not always clear. The case of cholestero'
is a perfect demonstration of this. Unfortunately, with
so many people's health and even lives at stake, ther
nothing funny about confusion and lack of clarity.

Cholesterol is a fatty substance produced by th
liver and is used to help perform thousands of bo
functions—so many that it is actually a key to l'
body uses it to
help build cell
membranes,
the covering of
nerve sheaths,
and much of the
brain. It is also
important in hormone production: wit'
the body would not have adequate le'
one, estrogen, progesterone or cortis'

*The total amount
cholesterol in the b
not by itself a dete'
of heart hea'*

a
it
n
va
An
the
mak
it do
coun
resear

With all the talk about the pro'
cholesterol, one startling fact stan
who have heart attacks have nor

American Heart Association and a professor of medicine at the University of Colorado School of Medicine in Aurora, sums up the finding this way: "HDL levels are related to risk, but that doesn't mean that raising HDL is beneficial."

Harvard Medical School research on this subject identified a gene variant that is found in about 2.6% of the population and is associated with elevated HDL levels: people with the variant have levels that average about six points higher than people without it. The researchers looked for the variant in about 21,000 people who had experienced heart attacks and 95,000 people with no heart-attack history. They found that people with the variant did indeed have higher HDL levels, but did *not* have lower susceptibility to heart attacks.

Statins lower LDL, but they do not lower it selectively, by targeting the dangerous oxidized form.

Researcher Sekar Kathiresan, MD, of Harvard Medical School and Massachusetts General Hospital, said, "The expectation was that the people who carried this genetic variant would have a lower heart attack risk, but that is not what we found."

Genes and Risk

A second study had similar results: it involved 14 more-common gene variants also associated with HDL. Again, the researchers found no evidence that the variants had a direct, protective role in heart-attack risk.

Some doctors continue to use niacin to raise HDL, but that whole protocol is now in question, and niacin's own side effects make it less than optimal for treating cardiac risk. And searches for new drugs to raise HDL, which have gone on for many years, have not gone well. For example, in 2006, Pfizer abandoned its experimental HDL-boosting drug *torcetrapib* because trials showed an increase in heart-attack and stroke risk among users.

"What we do know is that lowering LDL has a big impact on risk," says Dr. Eckel, "so the take-home message remains, 'Get those LDL numbers down.'" And that is certainly an endorsement of statins for many people.

> *"Lowering LDL has a big impact on risk."*
>
> —Robert Eckel, M.D.

Eli Farhi, MD, an assistant professor of cardiology at the University at Buffalo School of Medicine and Biomedical Sciences, agrees that "statins clearly decrease one's chance" of having a heart attack or stroke—but the amount of the decrease depends on how great your risk was in the first place. If your risk of heart attack in the next 10 years is relatively low—doctors do not all agree on a number, but 10% or so is generally considered reasonable—then statin use is of less value than if your risk is, say, 50%.

Here at last is something you can check for yourself—and a number that highlights the difficulty of deciding what to do about cholesterol. The National Cholesterol Education Program of the National Heart, Lung and Blood Institute has developed a simple calculator that anyone can use for free to assess cardiac risk. You can find it at the NHLBI Web site.

To use the calculator, you need to know your total cholesterol, HDL cholesterol and systolic blood pressure—the top number. Fill in the information and click on "calculate your 10-year risk" to receive a percentage likelihood that someone with your numbers will have a heart attack within 10 years—and suggestions on how your risk can be reduced.

Then—this is where it gets interesting—change some numbers and redo the calculation. You will find that a significant reduction in total cholesterol, say from 240 to 180, which is a 25% drop, will not make nearly as big a difference in risk as changing certain other numbers.

> **Example:** A 64-year-old nonsmoking man with cholesterol of 240—certainly high enough for most doctors to prescribe a statin—and HDL of 40, low enough to confirm a statin prescription, with slightly elevated systolic blood pressure of 140, has a 17% chance of a heart attack within 10 years. Reduce the cholesterol number to 180—a 25% drop—and his risk falls to 14%, which is a smaller decline: 17%.

> But drop the man's age to 54, leaving his cholesterol at 240 and all other numbers the same, and his heart-attack risk is just 11%, falling to 7%—a 36% drop—if cholesterol drops to 180. So: being younger, and reducing cholesterol at a younger age, will have far more effect on heart-attack risk.

Being female drops risk even more—much more. Return to the example of the 64-year-old with cholesterol of 240, but this time use female rather than male for gender. Now the risk of a heart attack within 10 years is just 5%, which is very low by any standards. Reducing cholesterol to 180 for this woman, which is still a 25% decline, lowers risk to 4%—a 20% drop from a number that is already very low.

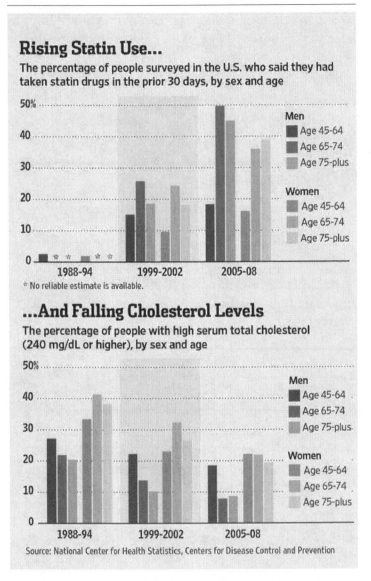

Rising Statin Use...

The percentage of people surveyed in the U.S. who said they had taken statin drugs in the prior 30 days, by sex and age

Men
- Age 45-64
- Age 65-74
- Age 75-plus

Women
- Age 45-64
- Age 65-74
- Age 75-plus

1988-94   1999-2002   2005-08

* No reliable estimate is available.

...And Falling Cholesterol Levels

The percentage of people with high serum total cholesterol (240 mg/dL or higher), by sex and age

Men
- Age 45-64
- Age 65-74
- Age 75-plus

Women
- Age 45-64
- Age 65-74
- Age 75-plus

1988-94   1999-2002   2005-08

Source: National Center for Health Statistics, Centers for Disease Control and Prevention

Then drop the woman's age to 54 for some truly significant changes: now, with cholesterol of 240, her heart-attack risk is only 3%, and reducing cholesterol to 180 drops it to 1%, which is as low as the calculator goes.

So whatever concerns there are regarding cholesterol, what is clear is that to avoid heart attack, it is better to be younger and female than older and male. There is not much that statins can do about that.

The fact is that the picture of cholesterol's involvement in cardiac disease is by no means clear. Countries including Austria, Belgium and France have high saturated-fat consumption and high average cholesterol levels, but low levels of heart disease; countries including Georgia, Ukraine and Croatia consume low amounts of saturated fat and have low average cholesterol levels, but have high heart-disease mortality rates.

An intriguing study published in the journal *Circulation* found that average cholesterol levels seem to rise and fall along with their countries' economies and ease of access to quality health care. Rates of total high cholesterol varied widely, ranging from 73% in Bulgaria to 24% in Finland; rates were especially high in Lithuania, Romania, Ukraine, Hungary and Russia, in addition to Bulgaria. All these countries scored relatively low in terms of their economies and health systems.

The United States' rate of people with elevated cholesterol levels was similar to that of other developed countries: Australia, Canada, Finland, Israel and the United Kingdom. The study's lead author, Elizabeth Magnuson, ScD, Director of Health Economics and Technology Assessment at Saint Luke's Mid America Heart Institute in Kansas City, Missouri, commented that differences in nations' rates of high cholesterol "may be due to differences in clinical guidelines, as well as whether and the extent to which guidelines are followed and specific initiatives are effectively implemented," making management of heart disease difficult.

Dark Side of Low Cholesterol

That is, if anything, an understatement. As far back as 1992, just five years after statins became widely available, *The New York Times* was reporting on the "dark side to having especially low cholesterol levels," citing studies showing people with very low levels of cholesterol in their blood to be more likely to die in later years from suicide, homicide, strokes, certain cancers, liver disease and lung disease—with deaths from these causes rising so quickly that the mortality rate for those with low cholesterol levels equals the rate for people with very high cholesterol levels, who are likely to die from heart disease.

Stephen Hulley, MD, a heart disease researcher at the University of California in San Francisco, said at the time that this constituted "a very serious and disconcerting set of observations," while Antonio Gotto, MD, a cardiologist at Baylor College of Medicine in Houston and a leader in the movement to change the American diet to lower the average cholesterol level, said, "We are moving to a position of policy where we would be lowering the cholesterol levels of millions of asymptomatic people and keeping their levels low for a lifetime. It behooves us therefore to be sure we are not doing any harm."

People with very low levels of cholesterol in their blood are more likely to die in later years from suicide, homicide, strokes, certain cancers, liver disease and lung disease.

"First, do no harm" is the famous foundation of medical-school teaching, often referred to as the beginning of the Hippocratic Oath despite the fact that the words do not actually appear there—although the oath includes a similar promise: to abstain from doing harm. But it has proved deucedly difficult to know when one is doing harm and when one is doing good when it comes to cholesterol and the overall management of cardiovascular disease. David H. Newman, MD, an emergency physician and Director of Clinical Research at Mt. Sinai School of Medicine in New York City, told *The Saturday Evening Post* that "cholesterol levels are actually a fairly weak predictor of who will have a heart attack," noting that this fact "has shocked everyone." And that "everyone" does not only refer to doctors—it is shocking information for patients, too, since at this point "everyone knows" the dangers of high cholesterol. What "everyone knows" is simply not true.

Nor is this the only shock. Information indicating that lower cholesterol does not neces-

> *"Cholesterol levels are actually a fairly weak predictor of who will have a heart attack."*

sarily lead to a longer life has been around for decades. A study published in July 1992 in *Archives of Internal Medicine* involved some 350,000 healthy middle-aged men, 6% of whom had very low total cholesterol levels. According to lead researcher James Neaton, MD, of the University of Minnesota, and his colleagues, the men in that 6% had hardly any heart disease 12 years later, and their death rate *from heart attacks* was about half that of men with cholesterol levels of 200 to 239. But the men in the 6% were *more* likely to die of *other* diseases. They were twice as likely to have an intracranial hemorrhage, three times as likely to have liver cancer, twice as likely to die of lung disease—an association that, unsurprisingly, was strongest among the men who smoked—twice as likely to kill themselves, and five times as likely to die of alcoholism.

David Jacobs, MD, an epidemiologist at the University of Michigan, said at the time that the whole topic made him very uncomfortable: "We as scientists don't know exactly how to react to these findings." He was talking about some of his own that, like those reported in *Archives of Internal Medicine*, were genuinely unsettling.

A study of 170,000 men and 120,000 women in various countries showed a consistently increased mortality rate from low cholesterol levels.

Dr. Jacobs' study, published in the journal *Circulation*, studied 170,000 men and 120,000 women in various countries and showed a consistently increased mortality rate from low cholesterol levels. It also showed that men and women were equally at risk of dying from a variety of causes when their cholesterol levels are low.

The editor of *Circulation* at the time, Michael H. Criqui, MD, an epidemiologist at the University of California at San Diego, pointed out that Dr. Jacobs' study—like previous studies, including Dr. Neaton's—showed that the real mortality problem occurs when cholesterol levels drop below 160, and that in any case the data do not prove cause and effect: does low cholesterol cause mortality from non-cardiac causes, or do people with non-cardiac diseases tend to have low cholesterol?

Low Cholesterol and Violence

All these years later, there is no certain answer to the question, and plenty of researchers are still working on it. One of the top ones, Beatrice A. Golomb, MD, PhD—who, like Dr. Criqui, is based at the University of California at San Diego—reported in *Annals of Internal Medicine* that people with low cholesterol have demonstrated increased violent behaviors, and more die violent deaths. In fact, she said that men who were receiving cholesterol-lowering therapy, but didn't have heart disease, died violently at rates she labeled as excessive. On the other hand, a group of Stanford scientists concluded that putting more people on cholesterol-lowering drugs, even if the individuals did not fall under current treatment guidelines, would help lower the economic and health burden of heart disease.

So there remains plenty of confusion about cholesterol, as this brief survey of arguments and research shows. If doctors who have devoted their careers to cardiovascular issues and to the study of cholesterol cannot say definitively just how important cholesterol levels—and levels of the lipids that move cholesterol around—are for heart health, how can patients possibly figure out what they should do?

One reasonable approach would be to turn to some of the most respected treatment centers in the United States and get their clinicians' opinions on cardiovascular self-protection.

9

The View
from Cleveland

Two of the most respected medical centers in the
United States are the Cleveland Clinic in Ohio
and the Mayo Clinic in Rochester, Minnesota,
with branches in Florida and Arizona. The medical
skill of the doctors and other health-care professionals
at these clinics, the team approach to treatment that
both organizations espouse, and the emphasis on disease prevention and—when a disease cannot be prevented—catching the condition early and dealing with
it in its most-treatable stage, have combined to make
the Cleveland Clinic and Mayo Clinic into paradigms
of the best modern medical care. Both have frequently
been cited by politicians of all stripes and by various
medical and health-oriented organizations as potential
models for the entire health-care system in the United
States.

Given the complexity of the issues surrounding
statins, cholesterol, and heart disease prevention and
treatment, and the need for patients to get understandable, plainspoken explanations of the factors involved
in cardiovascular conditions and the best approaches
for people to follow in order to protect their health, it
makes sense to consult the Cleveland Clinic and Mayo
Clinic for their views on the complex and interrelated
subjects—and their treatment protocols.

The Cleveland Clinic offers its analyses and commentaries at a number of interlaced Web sites. There is a great deal of information at these sites—far more than most people will easily be able to absorb in a reasonable *The Cleveland Clinic and Mayo Clinic are paradigms of the best modern medical care.* time—and there is inevitably some overlap of material among them. But a careful reading of the relevant presentations makes it possible to present what could be called the Cleveland Clinic overview of heart disease, cholesterol and statins.

The Basics of Cholesterol

It starts with a straightforward explanation of cholesterol, noting that your body needs it to make hormones, skin oils, digestive juices and vitamin D, but that too much cholesterol is a major risk factor for heart disease—particularly when there is too high a level of LDL, low density lipoprotein. The clinic does not discuss the differing types of particles within LDL cholesterol, but gives a good basic overview that introduces the subject clearly and intelligently. Then it explains that the body makes some cholesterol on its own, while some comes from foods—animal products only, since foods from plants do not contain cholesterol. And then the Cleveland Clinic notes that cholesterol cannot travel in the blood on its own but is carried by special proteins, with combinations of cholesterol and protein carriers being called lipoproteins.

The clinic simplifies by saying that there are two types of lipoproteins, low-density lipoproteins (LDLs, or "bad" cholesterol) and high-density lipoproteins (HDLs, or "good" cholesterol). There are actually five types of lipoproteins: HDL and LDL are the two most often discussed, but there are also very-low-density lipoproteins or VLDL, intermediate-density lipoproteins or IDL, and chylomicrons. But as introductory material, this explanation is helpful.

Then the Cleveland clinic comes up with a useful image: "Think of LDLs as delivery trucks and HDLs as garbage trucks. LDLs pick up cholesterol from the liver and deliver it to cells. HDLs remove excess cholesterol from the blood and take it to the liver."

This truck metaphor is a nice way of simplifying the bodily functions of HDL and LDL, although it *is* a simplification. For the basic purpose of understanding the difference between the two most commonly discussed types of lipoproteins, it is fine.

So what, then, is the problem with cholesterol? The Cleveland Clinic says that the body produces plenty of cholesterol on its own to keep people healthy, but the additional cholesterol from foods in the typical American diet can lead to high blood-cholesterol levels and then to heart disease. The excess cholesterol, deposited in arteries, joins with other substances to produce the thick, hard deposit called plaque—and when plaque builds up, the result is atherosclerosis, often called "hardening of the arteries." The danger is that plaque can narrow the passage inside the artery, reducing the flow of blood to the heart muscle.

"Think of LDLs as delivery trucks and HDLs as garbage trucks."

One thing that is not said here is that, because most cholesterol in the body is produced by the body itself, the effect of dietary change on cholesterol levels may not be significant unless a person eats a particularly unhealthful diet—and a lot of food. Another thing that is not mentioned here is that when blood flow to the heart muscle drops below a certain level, the result is cardiac pain, cardiac insufficiency, and possibly a heart attack. That is the danger against which lifestyle decisions and medications such as statins are designed to guard.

Cholesterol-Level Factors

The Cleveland Clinic points out that high total cholesterol does not always indicate an increased risk for heart disease. But what determines a healthful cholesterol level? The Cleveland Clinic's list includes your HDL level compared with your LDL level; your total cholesterol level; the number of risk factors for heart disease that you have; your age and activity level; and your current health status. This is a simple and comprehensive list.

As for what the risk factors for heart disease are, the Cleveland Clinic says that in addition to cholesterol levels, they include diabetes, smoking, high blood pressure,

> "Plaque can...pinch off the flow of blood to the heart muscle."

obesity, a sedentary lifestyle, a family history of heart disease, and age—45 years and older for men, 55 and older for women.

And what should people concerned about cholesterol do to lower it? Initially, the Cleveland Clinic specifically recommends only lifestyle changes: eat fewer fats and fried foods; consume unsaturated fats when possible; eat fish and poultry more often than red meat; consume no more than seven ounces a day, total, of meat, fish, poultry and low-fat cheeses; exercise regularly; if you smoke, quit; if you are overweight, lose the excess pounds; eat more soluble fiber; and have no more than three egg yolks per week.

The Cleveland Clinic's discussion of statins comes separately, beginning with an explanation that some 81 million American adults are living with CVD, cardiovascular disease—hypertension, coronary heart disease, heart failure, stroke and/or congenital cardiovascular heart defects. And more than 17 million people with CVD have coronary heart disease, a buildup of fat—that is, atherosclerotic plaque—in the walls of the arteries around the heart. Coronary heart disease, the clinic points out, is the number one cause of death in the United States.

Then the Cleveland Clinic discusses statins, weighing in decisively on the side of those who believe they are an important primary-prevention treatment. The clinic states that statins are important for primary prevention—helping prevent coronary heart disease in patients without a history of it. And it says statins are also important for people who are at high risk of developing cardiovascular disease, such as patients with diabetes, or who have already had some form of the dis-

Excess cholesterol, deposited in arteries, joins with other substances to produce the thick, hard deposit called plaque.

ease—such as a heart attack, stroke, transient ischemic attack or TIA, angioplasty, coronary artery stent placement or peripheral vascular disease. In other words, the clinic comes down squarely in favor of statins for both primary and secondary prevention.

The clinic describes statins as the first-line treatment of choice for patients with high cholesterol and those diagnosed with coronary heart disease. And it says statins have additional benefits beyond lowering cholesterol levels: they also help the lining of the blood vessels work better, make atherosclerotic plaques more stable and therefore less likely to do damage, reduce the amount of inflammation and damage done to cells through oxidation, and lower blood-clot risk by keeping blood platelets from clumping together.

These last observations are significant for enumerating effects of statins that are not always part of the arguments for and against the medicines. Indeed, some researchers now believe that statins' primary value lies in the extent to which they reduce inflammation, not in what they do to lower cholesterol.

Statin-Supporting Studies

The Cleveland Clinic cites several specific studies supporting the use of statins, then carefully notes that these potent medications are not without side effects such as muscle discomfort. The clinic says lower-dose or less-frequent statin use may help relieve myopathy, and that some patients benefit from Coenzyme Q-10— CoQ-10.

The Cleveland Clinic concludes its statin discussion by returning to the matter of lifestyle changes, and it gets quite specific about some recommendations, suggesting regular exercise of about an hour a day—more than many doctors and other organizations call for; better food choices; and

The Cleveland Clinic says statins have additional benefits beyond lowering cholesterol levels.

maintenance of a body mass index below 25. Furthermore, the clinic says that living healthfully also means
eating breakfast every day, weighing yourself at least
once a week and watching less than 10 hours of television weekly.

A separate discussion of statins, created by a group
of prominent Cleveland Clinic doctors writing as the
Beating Edge Team, actually celebrates the medications and advocates
them quite strongly:
"We're happy to lead the "We're happy to lead
cheers for a drug when the cheers for a drug
it's appropriate." when it's appropriate." These doctors say that even some people with
normal cholesterol should take statins. And yes, statins
have side effects, but the doctors say this is not a major
concern—because the risk of muscle aches, stiffness
and mild elevations in liver-function tests is both slight
and reversible

Furthermore, citing a study in *The Lancet,* the
Beating Edge Team says that taking statins could lower
the risk of heart disease by as much as 20% in people
who have *no* record of heart problems. This benefit,
team members say, is so great that it far outweighs the
statistical risks for rare adverse side effects, and suggests
that "statins perhaps ought to be prescribed much more
widely than they are already."

Well, that is certainly a
controversial statement—
the anti-statin forces are
as well entrenched as the
pro-statin ones, and neither
group seems likely to give
ground, since both believe

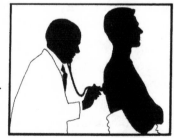

they have patient benefits in the forefront of their minds and recommendations. Notice that these Cleveland Clinic doctors specifically state that the side effects of statins are not only a slight risk but are also reversible—a

"Statins perhaps ought to be prescribed much more widely than they are already."

statement that anti-statin forces would strongly dispute, especially in the case of rhabdomyolysis.

Just how many people should be using statins? The Beating Edge Team doctors point out that nearly 40% of people who die of cardiovascular disease have few or none of the known risk factors. Therefore, they say that taking statins—according to the *Lancet* study—could save millions of lives of people who are not at obvious cardiovascular risk, especially people over age 50. But they then ask, reasonably, whether statins should be given to healthy people to prevent future heart disease—a significant bone of contention in the pro-and-con arguments about statins.

Their answer is that heart disease will affect 50% of people, and one-third will die from it. Therefore, says Stanley Hazen, MD, head of Preventive Cardiology at Cleveland Clinic, "we take a very aggressive approach toward statin use." Hazen says that statins are proven lifesavers, and adds that as a result, clinic doctors often recommend using them in people who might not otherwise be considered candidates for statin therapy based on more-conservative national guidelines. The patient's total risk profile is what matters, he says, in determining whether the patient should be on a statin.

The Beating Edge Team doctors say that the Cleveland Clinic has "been full of statin enthusiasts" since long before publication of the *Lancet* study. Making a lighthearted comment on a serious subject, the doctors say that "cardiologists jokingly recommend that statins ought to be put in the drinking water." Steven Nissen, MD, and A. Marc Gillinov, MD, both of Cleveland Clinic, say in their book *Heart 411* that they cannot endorse *that* idea—but they nevertheless strongly advocate statins because the bottom line is that these medications prevent heart attacks, prevent strokes, and save lives.

Not for Everybody

However, the doctors' enthusiasm is tempered by the reality that no medicine is suitable for use under all circumstances, by all people. Dr. Nissen specifically comments, "All medications have risks and we don't recommend statins for everyone." Specifically, there is no evidence that statins are beneficial for people at low cardiovascular-disease risk—and of course, every patient's personal and clinical profile is different, so each individual needs to speak with his or her doctor about the medications' risks and benefits in his or her particular circumstances.

That is, of course, an eminently reasonable recommendation, and one that every doctor will endorse, since none wishes to prescribe medications for patients other than his or her own. But as reasonable as it is, the statement may also be a recipe for frustration, since few individual doctors will be as well-informed—or as prominent in their fields—as those at the Cleveland Clinic. Indeed, many doctors as well as patients look to the Cleveland Clinic for help guiding them through the pluses and minuses of statin use and other tricky medical questions. They look to the Mayo Clinic as well, with equal hopefulness and attentiveness.

10

The Mayo Clinic's View

A visitor to the Mayo Clinic's Web site will likely be overwhelmed by the sheer amount of material available. The user-friendly site not only covers a huge variety of topics but also displays, along the left side, supplementary links to whatever material you happen to be looking at...and each link then displays its own links...and you can very easily have an Alice in Wonderland experience, falling down what seems to be an infinite rabbit hole of information and recommendations.

The material is carefully written to be easily understandable, but there is a *lot* of it—which of course makes sense when dealing with complicated medical matters, but which can frustrate anyone trying to take command of his or her health, or simply wanting to understand better what options there are and what risks accompany each one.

> *The Mayo Clinic's material is carefully written to be easily understandable, but there is* lot *of it.*

For example, there is a page—actually two pages—headlined "Statins: Are these cholesterol-lowering drugs right for you?" It would seem reasonable to turn to this entry for straightforward yes-or-no answers. But in fact, in addition to the two pages of material under that particular question, there is a left-hand column

that offers three related entries under the "alternative medicine" heading, one under "causes," two under
"definition," seven under "lifestyle and home remedies,"
one under "prevention," two under "risk factors," two
under "tests and diagnosis," and five under "treatments
and drugs." And every single one of the 23 discussions
under those headings connects to new material that
then has its *own* cross-references. To say this is a lot is a
vast understatement.

Nevertheless, the Mayo Clinic's material is out-
standing for the ease with which just about any information can be located—and the simplicity with which
complex subjects are presented. Overviews are easy to
come by, and anyone who wants to get really deeply
into a particular area of concern will find many, many
ways to do so.

Regarding statins, the Mayo Clinic reasonably
explains that the decision on whether or not you need
to be on a statin depends on your cholesterol level, but
not on that alone—other risk factors for cardiovascular
disease must also be taken into account. The clinic's
doctors point out that in addition to being effective in
reducing cholesterol, statins may have other possible
benefits, but many questions about them remain unan-
swered—whether they are right for everyone with high
cholesterol or only for some people; what the effects are
of taking a statin for decades; whether statins can help
prevent diseases other than cardiovascular disease; and
so forth. This is the sort of broad-brush view, with wide-
ranging questions, that the Mayo Clinic is particularly
adept at providing.

When to Use Statins

So—use a statin or no? Again, the clinic emphasizes that whether an individual needs to be on a statin depends on his or her cholesterol level and on other risk factors for cardiovascular disease. It makes sense to start by knowing what high-cholesterol numbers are—total cholesterol level of 240 milligrams per deciliter or higher, and/or low-density lipoprotein cholesterol level of 130 mg/dL or above—because those are levels at which many doctors will recommend that patients begin to take statins.

"If the only risk factor you have is high cholesterol, you may not need medication."

But not all doctors will automatically prescribe statins for people with these numbers, because "if the only risk factor you have is high cholesterol, you may not need medication," since your heart-attack and stroke risk could, taken as a whole, be low. After all, high cholesterol is just one of a number of cardiovascular risk factors.

Most of the risk factors should by now be familiar, but the Mayo Clinic includes two that do not always show up on other lists: family history of high cholesterol or cardiovascular disease, and peripheral artery disease, which is a narrowing of the arteries in your arms, legs or neck.

And, like other medical institutions and doctors in general, the Mayo Clinic points out that "lifestyle changes are essential for reducing your risk of heart disease," whether or not you take a statin. The Mayo Clinic says that those changes fall into four categories:

stop smoking; eat a diet low in fat, salt and cholesterol, even though dietary cholesterol is not the body's
primary source; exercise most days of the week, for 30
minutes per session; and manage stress.

Other Mayo Clinic presentations get into details
about these categories and many other matters, but
the clinic's overview continues by telling patients that
statins are generally a long-term commitment, not a
short-term solution. This is
a point that everyone thinking about statins needs to
understand: once you begin
to use them, you will likely
continue doing so for the rest
of your life. It may seem logi-
cal that, once your cholesterol goes down, you can stop
taking a statin. But statins are not like aspirin, acetaminophen and other fever reducers, to be taken when
the numbers go up and stopped when they are lower. A
prescription for statins is usually a lifetime decision—
cardiovascular risk factors that are reduced by a statin
will likely return to dangerous levels if you stop taking
the medication.

"Lifestyle changes are essential for reducing your risk of heart disease."

—Mayo Clinic

There is, however, an exception: making significant
dietary changes or losing a lot of weight. If you make
and stick to these substantial lifestyle alterations, you
may be able to lower your cholesterol without continuing to take a statin—but these are big changes that
many people find very difficult. And in any case, the
Mayo Clinic warns, you should not make significant
changes to your lifestyle or any changes to your medications without talking to your doctor first.

Side Effects

As for statins' side effects, the Mayo Clinic divides them into two categories. The more-likely ones include muscle and joint aches, nausea, diarrhea and constipation. Less common but potentially more serious are liver damage, which can potentially be serious enough to require the cessation of statin use; myopathy (muscle pain) and the far more serious muscle breakdown (rhabdomyolysis); increased blood glucose levels, which are a small risk but could lead to development of type 2 diabetes; and such neurological side effects as memory loss or confusion—which, if they do occur, stop in patients who stop taking statins.

"Statins could also have benefits that help prevent diseases that aren't related to your heart health."

In all cases, the Mayo Clinic says to talk to your doctor—but not stop taking statins on your own—if you notice any unusual symptoms or difficulties while taking statins. However, the clinic does not point out that side effects may take a long time to show up—one reason patients and doctors alike are not always sure whether they *are* side effects of statins. Nevertheless, the Mayo Clinic's reminder to tell your doctor about any unusual symptoms is thoughtful and well-considered. So is its recommendation to check whether statins could interact with any other drugs or supplements—prescription or over-the-counter—that you may be taking.

One thing the Mayo Clinic does very well is to remind patients, again and again, of how individual-

Atorvastatin

ized statin treatment, like other medical treatments, needs to be, pointing out that because of genetic differences, the type of statin, its dose, and the potential combination of statins with other cholesterol-lowering drugs can vary from person to person. There are a lot of possible variations—a bewildering array of them, in fact. For some patients, adding *ezetimibe*, sold as Zetia®, to statins can drop LDL levels further than statins alone. For others, statins may be combined with niacin; in still other cases, fish-oil supplements, or fibric-acid agents such as *gemfibrozil* (Lopid) may be indicated. And then there are combination medicines such as Simcor® and TriCor® that include both a specific statin and niacin. The possible drugs and drug combinations go on and on, and must be carefully individualized for each patient—which of course requires close and ongoing consultation with your doctor to determine what makes the most sense for you, how well a particular regimen is working once it is begun, and how and when to change it if it is not producing the desired results.

Tons of Information

Anyone whose head is spinning at this point can be readily forgiven: the Mayo Clinic provides detail and background that likely go well beyond what patients have heard before. For example, the clinic discusses statins' anti-inflammatory properties, saying that these medicines' potentially far-reaching effects may involve the brain and organs throughout the body as well as the heart and blood vessels.

Statins may help stabilize blood-vessel linings, which would make accumulated plaque deposits less likely to rupture and cause a heart attack. Statins can also help relax blood vessels; that lowers blood pressure. And statins can reduce the risk of formation of blood clots. For

Side effects of statins may take a long time to show up.

all these reasons, the clinic explains, some doctors now prescribe statins before and after coronary artery bypass surgery or angioplasty—and also put patients on them after certain kinds of strokes.

Furthermore, the Mayo Clinic notes that statins may help prevent non-cardiovascular diseases—including arthritis, some forms of cancer, dementia, Alzheimer's disease and kidney disease—although these uses are not universally accepted and further research is needed.

But to go back to statins' primary use: what if a statin does *not* help you lower your cholesterol satisfactorily? The Mayo Clinic says that your doctor may add other medications to a statin—or may suggest that you make more lifestyle changes to help lower your cardiovascular risk. And what, specifically, might such changes entail? The Mayo Clinic does a particularly good job of getting down to specifics about these issues, as we shall see.

11

Lifestyle with Mayo

The Mayo Clinic is unique among major medical institutions in the United States for the extent of its focus on lifestyle and so-called "alternative" approaches to health in addition to medical ones that use the traditional prevent-and-cure-disease model. Excerpts from its many free offerings about healthful living show the attentiveness with which the Mayo Clinic addresses issues that go beyond diagnosing disease and eradicating it with medications, surgery and other standard medical practices.

There is one stylistic irritant in its material, but it is easy to get used to: the clinic often calls for "healthy" living, although that is not quite what the doctors mean—they are actually suggesting that you live a *healthful* life, one that is good for you, in order to have a *healthy* body, one that functions optimally.

The Mayo Clinic carefully avoids advocacy of statins *or* insistence on avoiding them if possible.

> *The Mayo Clinic carefully avoids advocacy of statins or insistence on avoiding them if possible. Instead, its doctors take a middle ground.*

Instead, its doctors take a middle ground, saying that while you can reduce cholesterol with medications, you can also try doing so by improving elements of your lifestyle. In fact, they say that even if you already take statins, lifestyle modifications can improve the medications' cholesterol-lowering effect.

First of All

The first Mayo Clinic recommendation is to lose excess weight, since "even just a few" extra pounds can raise cholesterol levels, while losing 5% to 10% of your body weight can help significantly reduce them. Then the clinic's doctors, unlike many others, address the all-important but rarely considered psychological elements of living in a way that is better for your health, telling people to be sure to consider their individual challenges to weight loss—and ways to overcome them. Among their examples: someone who eats when bored or frustrated can take a walk instead; someone who picks up fast food for lunch every day can pack something more healthful at home and bring it to work; someone who usually sits in front of the TV and snacks can put out a bowl of carrot sticks instead of potato chips.

The clinic also suggests that people avoid eating mindlessly and unthinkingly—instead, take time to enjoy food rather than gobbling it down. As for exercise, it does not always have to be carefully planned or associated with special equipment or a gym membership—many people can add physical activity to their daily routines easily, for example by using the stairs instead of taking the elevator at work. The clinic's very sensible bottom line is to think carefully about what you currently eat—and your current level of physical activity—and slowly work in changes.

Despite the moderate and reasonable language, all this is easier said than done, but the fact that the Mayo Clinic *does* say it is important. And the clinic then gets specific about the types of foods to eat in order to protect your heart. It urges getting less than 7% of daily calories from saturated fat—opting instead for lean meat and low-fat dairy products; and avoiding trans fats, found in fried foods and commercial baked goods, altogether—one thing that has become easier since many manufacturers have, on their own or under pressure, reduced their use of trans fats or stopped utilizing them completely.

Although cholesterol from food is not the primary source of cholesterol in the body, the Mayo Clinic nevertheless recommends limiting it—to 300 milligrams a day, or 200 mg/day if you have heart disease or diabetes. This means avoiding, or cutting way back on, consumption of organ meats, egg yolks and whole-milk products. The clinic also urges consuming more whole grains (in breads, pasta and flour, for example), and increasing consumption of fruits and vegetables—but not overdoing the use of *dried* fruit, which tends to have more calories than fresh. And the clinic recommends consuming more foods that are high in omega-3 fatty acids, substances that can help lower LDL—which means eating more of certain kinds of fish (such as salmon and mackerel) and making omega-3-rich walnuts, almonds and flaxseeds part of your diet *without* increasing your total calorie intake.

A Big Change for Many

These eating suggestions may represent a significant change for many people; and there is nothing particularly revolutionary about them—many doctors and organizations advocate essentially the same dietary approach. But the Mayo Clinic provides some useful specificity, such as the recommendations to keep saturated fat to 7% or less of daily calories and to limit dietary cholesterol to 300 mg or less—or 200 mg or less under some conditions. Dietary cholesterol is not the body's major source, but people who consume a large amount of cholesterol-containing food can raise their cholesterol levels through food consumption, so limiting intake makes sense.

Showing its understanding of psychological impediments to making lifestyle changes, the Mayo Clinic urges people to exercise on *most* days of the week, and adds, "Just be sure that you can keep up the changes you decide to make." Among physical activities that the clinic recommends are taking a brisk walk during lunch hour, riding a bike to work instead of driving, swimming laps, or playing a favorite sport. Since it can be difficult to

"Just be sure that you can keep up the changes you decide to make."

stay motivated on your own, the clinic suggests finding an exercise buddy or joining an exercise group. And it points out that *any* activity is helpful—just taking the stairs instead of the elevator at work, or doing a few situps while watching television, can make a difference if you do it regularly.

The Mayo Clinic offers one obvious lifestyle recommendation and one that may be surprising. The obvious one is to stop smoking. The one that may surprise people is to drink alcohol in moderation—if you already drink—because moderate alcohol use has been linked with higher levels of HDL cholesterol. However, the clinic says if you do *not* already drink, don't start, since the benefits that have been discovered are not strong enough to recommend alcohol consumption for anyone who does not already drink. As for what constitutes moderate alcohol consumption, the Mayo Clinic defines it as up to one drink a day for all healthy women and healthy men older than age 65, and up to two drinks daily for healthy men ages 65 and younger. *Moderate* consumption is key, because drinking too much alcohol can lead to serious health problems, including high blood pressure, heart failure and stroke.

Despite all its focus on lifestyle changes, the Mayo Clinic acknowledges that such changes alone may not be enough to lower cholesterol levels; and that brings us back to the use of statins and other medications—which the clinic points out should be used in addition to lifestyle improvements, not as a substitute for them.

Dietary Matters

The lifestyle change that many people find the most complex involves eating, since the typical American diet is quite different from the one recommended by the Mayo Clinic and other organizations. Mayo Clinic doctors understate things when they call their recommendations "a few simple tweaks to your diet"—the changes are by no means simple for people who have eaten very differently for decades—but the doctors do a good job of explaining why they recommend what they call the top five foods to lower cholesterol numbers.

The first food—really a food group—is oatmeal, oat bran and other high-fiber foods, because the soluble fiber in oatmeal (also found in apples, barley, kidney beans, pears and prunes) reduces LDL. The reason these foods are important is that soluble fiber—an amount of five to 10 grams a day, or more, is recommended—can reduce the absorption of cholesterol into the bloodstream. The clinic suggests people "mix it up a little" by combining various high-fiber foods, such as bananas plus cereal made with oatmeal or oat bran. This "mixing it up" is psychologically important to prevent people from feeling that they are, in effect, consuming bowls of medicine rather than good food.

Mix several good-for-you, good-tasting foods together so you do not feel you are eating bowls of medicine.

The second food, or food group, consists of fish and other foods containing omega-3 fatty acids—at least two servings a week, baked or grilled to avoid adding unhealthful fats. Ground flaxseeds and canola oil can also provide omega-3s, and so can supplements—but supplement users who do not like fish must be careful to eat lean meat or vegetables instead." Again, the idea is to provide a general recommendation and then alternatives, so people do not feel put-upon and find themselves not enjoying their meals—which is a recipe for returning to less-healthful eating habits.

The third food group that the Mayo Clinic focuses on is nuts—specifically ones such as walnuts, almonds, hazelnuts, peanuts, pecans, some pine nuts and pistachio nuts—which can help lower blood cholesterol. The recommendation here, though,

Nuts are beneficial if you consume the right amount—which is a small amount.

depends highly on consuming the correct—which is to say small—amount: one-and-a-half ounces a day, which is a small handful. And the clinic warns that it is important to make sure that the nuts are not salted or coated with sugar. In fact, the reference to sugar is only one part of the issue with nuts: all nuts are high in calories, and it is very easy to eat too many. The Mayo Clinic's suggestion is to replace foods high in saturated fat with nuts, for example by adding walnuts or almonds to a salad instead of tossing in cheese, meat or croutons. Once again, that is a simple, practical solution that may make nuts more appealing to people who are not fond of them. Adding some crunch to a salad makes the salad itself more palatable to many people.

Oils and Sterols

The fourth and fifth foods that the Mayo Clinic mentions are not foods that you sit down and consume as a main course or even a side dish. They are olive oil and foods with added plant sterols or stanols. Olive oil contains antioxidants that can lower LDL and raise HDL, but no one drinks it by the glass. Nor do you have to; nor should you; the Mayo Clinic simply suggests using about two tablespoons of olive oil a day in place of other fats in your diet—for example, by sautéing vegetables in it, adding it to a marinade or mixing it with vinegar as a salad dressing.

Olive oil contains antioxidants that can lower LDL and raise HDL.

The most-recommended oil is extra-virgin olive oil, which is less processed and therefore contains more heart-beneficial antioxidants. But olive oil, like nuts, is high in calories, so it is important to use it as a substitute for other oils that are less healthful—not simply to add it to your diet. And two tablespoons a day are plenty.

As for foods fortified with plant sterols or stanols, these are foods with added amounts of plant substances that help block cholesterol absorption. The Mayo Clinic says that margarines, orange juice and yogurt drinks with these additions can help reduce LDL by more than 10%; daily consumption needs to be at least two grams, which is about the amount in 16 ounces of plant-sterol-fortified orange juice.

Of course, this recommendation works only if you substitute fortified orange juice for your current brand—assuming you drink orange juice at all—and if the fortified brand does not cost significantly more than the regular one and tastes just as good to you. Since plant sterols and stanols do not seem to affect levels of triglycerides or HDL, they are not a major element in heart health, but may be helpful if you switch from other brands without fortification, such as standard margarines. Including these foods as one of the top five seems a touch over-zealous, but that is why people need to make their own decisions on lifestyle issues, even in the face of Mayo Clinic recommendations.

The point is that there are suggestions, ideas and recommendations aplenty out there, including many from very well-respected sources, but it is not possible for every recommendation to fit every individual—and that includes the standard recommendation to "talk to your doctor." Not all doctors are experts in heart health, and even those who are may not be experts in lifestyle changes, or dietary issues, or the potential interaction of statins with other medications, or a host of other matters. So where *does* someone turn for expertise in the widest possible variety of heart-health-related issues and ideas? Logic suggests the American Heart Association.

12

Have a Stronger Heart

Based in Dallas, the American Heart Association is a nonprofit organization that explains its reason for being straightforwardly: "Our mission is to build healthier lives, free of cardiovascular diseases and stroke." Obviously, cholesterol and statins are of major concern to the AHA. But unlike the Cleveland Clinic and Mayo Clinic, the AHA does not provide medical treatment—only information and research funding—so it avoids debates on significant clinical issues. However, because its mission involves presenting medical data to a wide variety of audiences, from the public to the medical community, it does offer overviews of significant clinical issues that can help provide a broad view of major cardiovascular concerns.

Like the Cleveland Clinic and Mayo Clinic, the AHA offers topic searches that take people to sets of articles; and within each article, there are hyperlinks to more information and/or other articles that focus on specific elements—for instance, a page called "Why Cholesterol Matters" includes links to "coronary heart disease," "heart attack," "stroke," "high blood pressure," "diabetes" and other topics, each of which contains a number of its own hyperlinks. It takes a fair amount of "clicking around" to get a full picture of any topic from the AHA, since individual articles generally cover only a small portion of any given topic and are designed to encourage readers to click through to specific areas in which they want more-in-depth discussions.

Neutrality

One key to AHA presentations is the care the organization takes to remain neutral on subjects that it deems best left for discussions with one's own doctor; thus, *"the AHA is not recommending or endorsing any specific products"*—emphasis in the original. However, the AHA does give its "take" on heart-attack prevention, emphasizing that patients should make diet and lifestyle changes, whether or not a doctor prescribes a cholesterol medication. The AHA breaks down lifestyle changes into just three categories: eating a good-for-your-heart diet, including lots of vegetables fruits, whole grains and high-fiber foods, plus fish at least twice a week; exercising for at least 30 minutes "more days than not"; and avoiding both tobacco smoke and, for nonsmokers, second-hand smoke.

The AHA uses heart-disease statistics to try to emphasize the extent of the disease very clearly, stating not only that cardiovascular disease is the No. 1 cause of death in *"2,200 Americans die of cardiovascular disease each day, an average of one death every 39 seconds."* the United States but also that "2,200 Americans die of cardiovascular disease each day, an average of one death every 39 seconds." That is a striking statistic that may help bring home the seriousness of heart disease to many people.

Many comments made by the AHA will be familiar to anyone who has read Cleveland Clinic and Mayo Clinic discussions, but the AHA often gives a slightly different slant to the information, as in the "one death every 39 seconds" example.

The specificity of AHA statistics extends to the organization's guidelines on consumption of fat. The AHA says to limit total fat intake to 25–35% of total calories each day, or even less; limit intake of saturated fat to 7% of total daily calories; keep trans fat intake to a minimum of less than 1% of total daily calories; and limit cholesterol intake from foods to less than 300 mg per day—or for those with coronary heart disease or an LDL level of 100 mg/dL or greater, to less than 200 milligrams a day.

The recommendations may sound familiar, but the AHA goes a step beyond them with the specific example of a sedentary female, 31–50 years old, who needs about 2,000 calories each day. Under AHA guidelines she should consume less than 14 grams of saturated fat, less than 2 grams trans fat and between 50 and 70 grams of total fat each day—with most fats coming

The American Heart Association suggests using a food diary to keep track of what you eat.

from sources of polyunsaturated and monounsaturated fats, such as fish, nuts, seeds and vegetable oils. And the AHA suggests using a food diary to keep track of what you eat—making it easier to know how healthful or unhealthful the foods you consume are.

The AHA provides brief answers to some questions that people may not think to ask their doctors. For example, just how are trans fatty acids, known by the acronym TFA, harmful? They tend to raise total blood cholesterol levels, says the AHA, and some scientists believe they raise cholesterol levels more than saturated fats do. But there are no standard methods of estimating the TFA content of foods—and it is hard to estimate how much you consume, especially long-term. Therefore, the AHA simply recommends consuming as little of these fats as possible.

Butter vs. Margarine

There are interesting sidelights in AHA articles that are worth exploring—for instance, speaking of fats, is butter better than margarine? Well, the AHA notes that some stick margarines contribute more trans fatty acids than unhydrogenated oils or other fats. But it adds that because butter is rich in both saturated fat and choles-terol, it is potentially a highly atherogenic food—that is, a food that causes the arteries to be blocked. In terms of margarines, the AHA points out that most come from vegetable fat and provide no dietary cholesterol; and the more liquid a margarine is the less hydrogenated it is and the lower its content of trans fatty acids. That means that tub and liquid margarines are the best for health.

Notice that, as with medication, the AHA stops short of actually making a recommendation—it does not really answer the "is butter better?" question, but provides infor-mation intended to help people make their own decisions.

And when it comes to medication, the AHA is similarly even-handed. It explains statins in a very few words, saying that they work in the liver to prevent the formation of cho-lesterol and are most effective at lowering LDL, but also have modest effects on lowering triglycerides and raising HDL.

"High cholesterol is one of the major controllable risk fac-tors for coronary heart disease, heart attack and stroke."

—American Heart Association

Likewise, the issue of statins' side effects, which looms large for many people, is treated briefly, with a comment that most side effects of statins are mild—and generally go away as your body adjusts. Muscle problems and liver abnormalities do occur, says the AHA, but they are rare—although your doctor may order regular liver function tests, to be on the safe side.

Helpfully, and in line with its intention of making medical information more approachable, the AHA provides a list of statins that are currently available in the United States. Those are atorvastatin (Lipitor®), fluvastatin (Lescol®), lovastatin (Mevacor® or Altoprev™), pravastatin (Pravachol®), rosuvastatin calcium (Crestor®), and simvastatin (Zocor®). Statins are also found in some combination medicines, including Advicor® (lovastatin + niacin), Caduet® (atorvastatin + amlodipine), and Vytorin™ (simvastatin + ezetimibe).

The issue of statins' side effects, which looms large for many people, is treated briefly.

The AHA points out that other medications are available for lowering cholesterol—niacin, for one, and also fibrates, which it notes are best at lowering triglycerides and in some cases increasing HDL levels, but are not very effective in lowering LDL. Fibrates, the AHA notes, may be used in combination with statins.

In addition, there are medicines called resins, also known as bile acid sequestrant or bile acid-binding drugs. These work in the intestines, promoting increased disposal of cholesterol. The body naturally uses cholesterol to make bile—an acid that is important in digestion. Resins bind to bile so it cannot be used; that causes the liver to make more bile; the more bile

it makes, the more cholesterol it uses; the more cholesterol being used by the liver, the less there is circulating
in the blood.

New Class of Drugs

The AHA also mentions selective cholesterol absorption inhibitors, relatively new cholesterol-lowering
medications that work by preventing the absorption of
cholesterol from the intestine. But none of the alternative classes of medicine is as effective, as well-known or
as widely used as statins; and as the AHA notes, some
of the medications, such as fibrates and niacin, are often
used as supplements to statins.

Although the AHA takes no position on specific
medications, it does take one on the issue of cholesterol—whether this substance is a major risk factor for
heart disease. Its viewpoint is an emphatic yes. "High
cholesterol is one of the major controllable risk factors
for coronary heart disease, heart attack and stroke. As
your blood cholesterol rises, so does your risk of coronary heart disease." And the more risk factors you have
in addition to high cholesterol—including, say, high
blood pressure or diabetes—the greater your risk. And
the greater the level of *each* risk factor, the greater your
overall risk.

The AHA, like other organizations, adds that the
risk is not only
total cholesterol
but also LDL,
which can mix
with other sub-
stances to form
the thick, hard

Pravastatin

deposits known as plaque—which can narrow arteries and make them less flexible, resulting in atherosclerosis. And if a clot forms and blocks a narrowed artery, that can lead to a heart attack or stroke.

So the AHA and prominent medical organizations agree on the importance of minimizing cholesterol—even if there is no absolute agreement on appropriate cholesterol, HDL and LDL levels for everyone. And they agree both on the importance

"Most of statins' side effects are mild and generally go away as your body adjusts."

—American Heart Association

of living a heart-healthful life and on the use of statins, with or without other medicines, when lifestyle alone is not enough to bring cholesterol under control.

13

Miraculous *and* Misguided

It turns out that statins deserve neither to be put on a pedestal nor to be demonized. The reality is that they are indeed miraculous medications—but some claims made for them are dubious, some are overstated, and their manufacturers and some of their proponents are guilty of advocating them more zealously than science and medicine can support, for conditions for whose use it is not clear that they have significant value.

It is important to understand that, while drug manufacturers certainly have an agenda that leads them to promote their medications for more uses by more people, this is not done out of evil or venality. Corporations are not public-service entities. They are profit-making and are responsible to their employees, and they are very major employers indeed: Pfizer has more than 100,000 employees, Merck 85,000, Hoffman-LaRoche 80,000, Johnson & Johnson 118,000, Glaxo-SmithKline 97,000, and so on. As public corporations, they are responsible to shareholders: people who hold a company's stock are the real owners of the company, even if the average individual owns only a minuscule amount of it.

Time is always running out for pharmaceutical companies as they invent new drugs, since their 20 years of patent protection begin when they apply for the patent for a new medicine—and that is many years before the drug is approved, if indeed it ever is: many drugs fail in clinical trials, and hundreds of millions of dollars invested in them are lost. Actual exclusive sales time for a many-hundred-million-dollar medication may be as little as seven years before generic-drug manufacturers, who have invested nothing in a medicine's research and development, get the right to manufacture it and sell it very inexpensively—a great system for patients, but one of constant pressure for the creators of new medications. Small wonder, then, that if a drug appears useful beyond what it was originally approved for, its manufacturer would like it to be taken by more people.

Time is always running out for pharmaceutical companies as they invent new drugs.

Where statins are concerned, this has led to the medications' use for primary prevention of heart attack and other cardiovascular events, not the secondary prevention for which statins were originally approved. And yes, their use for primary prevention is controversial and not accepted by all doctors or medical institutions. But that does not mean using them this way is wrong—just that there is disagreement about it. There is no vast conspiracy pushing statins inappropriately. In fact, now that a number of major statins are off patent and available in generic versions for about $50 per year, there is little financial incentive for any manufacturer to advocate vast expansion of their use.

Agendas in Conflict

And it is worth pointing out that just as drug manufacturers have an agenda where their medications are concerned, so do many of their most vocal opponents.

Naturopaths, proponents of holistic medicine, and other advocates of so-called alternative medical treatments are just that—advocates. They may believe strongly that their approach to bodily health, including cardiovascular health, is superior to that of the "medical establishment", which, in the case of statins, is by no means so monolithic

The evidence for even-more-widespread use of statins is not entirely clear and does not all point in one direction.

as alternative practitioners sometimes make it out to be. But this is their *belief*, not a statement of fact, and no matter how honestly and strongly it is held, it is a matter of faith as much as science.

Of course, it can be argued that doctors' belief in traditional approaches has a certain degree of faith inherent in it as well: although medicine is supposed to be scientific and evidence-based, the evidence for even-more-widespread use of statins is not entirely clear and does not all point in one direction. So doctors have to make decisions about which elements of the evidence they accept. And if they have not done the research themselves, their acceptance has an element of faith to it—based on their respect for particular researchers, for example, or for specific journals in which research has been published.

One of the greatest things about science is its willingness always to be wrong, to be disproved by new experiments—it is a tradition in scientific research to come up with a hypothesis for the outcome of an experiment and then work diligently to *disprove* it. Nevertheless, some doctors' attachment to statins is stronger than is fully justified by the studies that have been done to date.

So where does all this leave patients? There is simply no one-size-fits-all answer to that question. Consider: even a question as simple as how to relieve acute pain, as from a bump, bruise, minor cut, headache, etc., has no single answer—this is why some people take aspirin; some take acetaminophen, such as Tylenol®; some take naproxen, such as Aleve®; some take ibuprofen, such as Advil® or Motrin®; and so on. When it comes to a condition such as heart disease, which develops over many decades and manifests

Doctors have to make decisions about which elements of the evidence they accept.

differently in different people—and often very differently in men from the way it does in women—there are bound to be even more "right" answers. But not all answers will be right for all people; that is simply impossible.

The Healthful Life

The one subject on which all practitioners agree is that living more healthfully helps protect against heart disease.

Stay Healthy

1) Maintain an appropriate body weight, which usually means body mass index of 25 or below, although there is even some controversy about that;

2) Eat a diet containing lean meat, chicken and fish rather than substantial amounts of red meat and other foods that are high in saturated fat;

3) Exercise regularly—although, again, there is some argument as to whether regularly means daily, and some disagreement about the intensity of exercise that is most beneficial; and

4) Avoid smoking and stay away from secondhand smoke. For everyone who can do all these things, bravo.

But *not* everyone can do these things, at least without considerable stress associated with trying to make major lifestyle changes while also *living* one's life, which may include a job or more than one; family responsibilities to spouse or partner and to children, parents or both; and all the difficulties of everyday life. And the missing element in the list above is 5) reducing stress in one's life. Stress is a killer—the exact mechanism is not completely understood, but the hormonal imbalances associated with prolonged stress are definitely causative factors for heart disease and a host of other ailments. So to the extent that healthful living is stressful because it requires a major reorientation of a person's long-term lifestyle, attempts to live more healthfully can themselves contribute to cardiovascular disease.

We all take our lives into our own hands every day.

It is no good saying that this *shouldn't* be so, because it *is* so, and medicine, like science in general, needs to deal with realities, not utopias or wish lists.

So, again, where does this leave patients? It leaves them in the position of ultimately making their own decisions on subjects about which they cannot be fully informed, because there is so much information, and on which their professional consultants—doctors and other healthcare workers—do not necessarily agree. Patients are literally taking their lives in their own hands, whether they want to or not.

But this is not quite as dire a prospect as it may appear. We *all* take our lives into our own hands every day—every time we cross a street, drive an automobile, get onto an airplane, and yes, every time we choose what food to consume and decide whether to do a one-hour workout or spend the hour watching television. But when we do most everyday activities, we are not focusing directly on their health consequences, although maybe we should—another *should*. When we enter the office of a healthcare professional, though, we *are* looking directly at the ways in which we are responsible for our own lives; and this can be a daunting task.

The best thing that most of us can do for our own health is *educate ourselves*. It is not necessary—or, for that matter, possible—to understand as much about medicine as a doctor, or as much about alternative approaches as a naturopath. But it is both necessary and possible to ask practitioners questions that focus on your personal situation, that help you help them make the best possible recommendations for you as an individual. This applies to statin use and a great number of other elements of healthcare.

> *There is nothing wrong, and a great deal right, in asking questions to elicit information that will help you understand your personal risk factors.*

Throughout the time you spend in a doctor's office, you are hiring him or her—he or she works for you during that period. There is nothing wrong, and a great deal right, in asking questions to elicit information that will help you understand your personal risk factors, your options, and the consequences of your decisions on whether to use statins or any other medicine. The decisions *are* yours, not the doctor's. The consequences are yours, too. And that can be scary—but it does not have to be. The more you understand, the better—see the Chapter 15 for descriptions of clinical trials, so you understand what is and is not known about statins and other medicines when they are approved for use; for questions you can ask before beginning treatment with statins or other medicines; and for tests that you can discuss with your doctor to get the best possible sense of your own particular risk for cardiovascular disease.

And understand that research into statins and other medicines designed to fight cardiovascular disease is ongoing: there is no definitive answer to the many questions that remain about heart health and statin use. There is only a "what it is best for *me* to do *right now*" answer—a decision that everyone must determine on his or her own in con tation with doctors, and that may very well change as knowledge improves and scientific research brings new medications to market.

14

The Last Word
—for Now

I t would be a mistake to think that statins, for all the
good they do, have in any way "solved" the cardiovascular problems of the United States and the
rest of the world. The fact is that the nature of those
problems is not fully understood, and even when we
seem to be getting some things right in combating the
No. 1 killer in the United States, we are not always sure
why. Consider
one fascinating
bit of research
that appeared in
*The Journal of the
American Medi-
cal Association.*

*Between 1988 and 2010,
overall cholesterol levels in
the United States fell from
an average of 206 to an
average of 196.*

Scientists from the Division of Health and Nutrition
Examination Surveys of the National Center for Health
Statistics, part of the Centers for Disease Control and
Prevention, found that between 1988 and 2010, overall cholesterol levels in the United States fell from an
average of 206 to an average of 196, using the usual
measurement of milligrams per deciliter of blood. Average levels of LDL or "bad cholesterol" also dropped,
from 129 to 116, and average levels of HDL or "good
cholesterol" rose from 50.7 to 52.5.

This study, called "Trends in Lipids and Lipoproteins in US Adults, 1988-2010," offered excellent news for heart health—but its findings were deeply puzzling. These improvements in cardiovascular-disease markers occurred at exactly the same time that Americans were becoming more overweight and obese than ever—to the point that one-third of adult Americans were obese and even the state with the lowest percentage of obese adults, Colorado, had a 20% obesity rate.

Surprising Statistics

Theories abounded for this reported statistical improvement, but one fact is that no one really knows why it happened. Another fact is that the use of statins undoubtedly played a part: at the start of the study, 3% of adults were taking statins, and at the end, 15% were taking them. But a third fact is that adults *not* taking cholesterol-lowering medicines also showed improvement—so statins provide only a partial explanation of what happened.

What else may have been going on? Politicians were quick to claim credit: for example, New York City banned the use of trans fats in restaurants in 2007, and that could have resulted in more-healthful eating and reduced cholesterol levels; and political pressures of other kinds led to the reduction or elimination of trans fats in many foods, also possibly making people healthier even if their dietary choices were not necessarily more healthful. The reality is that no one really knows what happened or to what extent statins contributed to the positive news.

Less than a month after the appearance of the research about Americans' cholesterol levels, statins got another research boost, this one from Denmark, where scientists found that cancer patients taking statins were 15% less likely to die *of cancer or any other cause* than patients who were not taking statins. Statins as life preservers and prolongers? There had been some research on this before, but the Danish study—published in *The New England Journal of Medicine*—was a particularly intriguing one. The researchers looked only at what happened after cancer was diagnosed, not at whether statins might prevent it —a subject of considerable controversy. They analyzed 18,721 people over age 40 who were diagnosed with cancer in Denmark between 1995 and 2007—all of whom were taking statins regularly before their cancer was detected—and compared them with 277,204 people who had not taken statins regularly before beginning cancer treatments.

> *Cancer patients taking statins were 15% less likely to die of cancer or any other cause.*

Statins' benefits in cancer patients varied according to the type of cancer, from an 11% lower death rate for patients with pancreatic cancer to a 36% lower rate among cervical-cancer patients. The survival improvement was found clearly in 13 types of cancer and was less clear-cut in 14 other types. Of course, this does not make statins an alternative to chemotherapy or other forms of cancer treatment—something that the researchers were quick to point out—but it may make them worth considering in forms of cancer for which there are no good chemotherapy or other treatment options.

As in all research, the question of "why" is an intriguing one—and as in most research, it has no definitive answer. The best guess, from senior author

Stig Bojesen, MD, of the University of Copenhagen, was that statins' effectiveness in reducing blood cholesterol may deprive cancer cells of an important building block of cell membranes—that being what cholesterol is— and that this deprivation slows tumor growth. To learn more, further research is necessary—further research

Rosuvastatin

is *always* necessary. And there was one particularly intriguing finding of this study: cancer patients who took *less* than the recommended dose of a statin had a *higher* rate of survival than those who took higher doses. No one has any idea what that means.

On Beyond Statins

One thing that *is* **known** is that while all the intriguing aspects of statins continue to be investigated, intense research designed to make them far more effective, if not to replace them altogether, continues. There is, for example, an entirely new class of medicines called *PCSK9 inhibitors*—for *proprotein convertase subtilisin/ kexin type 9*—and early-stage and middle-stage investigations have shown that these experimental drugs reduce LDL by 40% to 70% within weeks. That is as big a reduction as the best statins achieve. But PCSK9 inhibitors appear to be usable *with* statins to lower cholesterol levels even further. If that proves out, it would be a major breakthrough affecting even people who do not get adequate cholesterol-lowering results from statins.

As Frederick Raal, MD, of the University of the Witwatersrand, in Johannesburg, South Africa, said after presenting one of several studies of PCSK9 inhibitors, "With these drugs, together with statins, you can get virtually everyone to the goal."

PCSK9 inhibitors may prove to be miraculous, as statins are, but they will not be as convenient as statins: they must be injected, usually every two to four weeks. And of course they are brand-new, brand-name, patent-protected drugs, and thus not nearly as inexpensive as generic statins. Nor can they be considered appropriate for all people with high cholesterol. But many major and mid-level drug companies are betting that they nevertheless present a huge market opportunity.

For instance, from Sanofi S.A. and Regeneron Pharmaceuticals comes a substance known as *SAR236553/ REGN727.* One study, published in *The New England Journal of Medicine,* found that patients given this drug plus

PCSK9 inhibitors may prove to be miraculous, as statins are, but they will not be as convenient as statins.

atorvastatin, the generic version of Lipitor®, had a 73% reduction in LDL levels—compared with just 17% for those taking the statin alone. That is an extraordinary difference.

Amgen has a PCSK9 inhibitor, too, known as *AMG 145,* and it too showed impressive LDL reductions when used with another drug—Zetia® or ezetimibe: the two medicines together lowered LDL by 63%, compared with a 15% reduction in patients using only Zetia®.

Pfizer, Roche, Eli Lilly and Alnylam all see PCSK9 medicines as the next frontier in cholesterol control. These drugs work differently from statins. The liver removes LDL from the blood after the LDL binds to receptors on the surface of liver cells and is taken into them. PCSK9 also binds to LDL receptors, destroying them along with the LDL. If PCSK9 does *not* bind to the receptors, they can return to the cell surface and remove additional cholesterol—and the PCSK9 inhibitors prevent that binding. Thus, they make liver removal of LDL more efficient, so the body itself removes more LDL from the bloodstream.

As fascinating and complex as the new frontiers-of-research studies are, and as interesting as it is to observe the scientific progress being made in supplementing or perhaps replacing statins in the future—all against a backdrop indicating that cholesterol levels in the U.S. appear to be dropping for reasons only partly related to the increase in statin usage—what understandably matters to most people is what to do right now, with the consensus knowledge and medications currently available.

The best answer is to make a decision based on as much information as you can gather. With statin use as with so many other subjects, knowledge is power. These drugs have proved miraculous for many people in many ways. But for *you* to use them may still be misguided. Statins can be, have been and are lifesavers. But they are not cure-alls, not excuses to live in ways that are bad for your body, with the drugs "taking care of" the effects of an unhealthful lifestyle. Despite the naysayers, there is generally nothing to be afraid of in using statins. Despite the most strident advocates, there is no reason to use them indiscriminately. Find a position between the two extremes—a position that is right for *you* and for *your* health—and statins can help you live a longer, healthier and much more satisfying life.

Make a decision based on as much information as you can gather.

15

Furthering Knowledge

Alexander Pope wrote, "A little learning is a dangerous thing," in *An Essay on Criticism* in 1709—meaning that a small amount of knowledge can mislead people into thinking they are more expert than they really are. However, a complete lack of knowledge can be even more dangerous than a little bit when it comes to medical matters, where life-extending and even lifesaving decisions need to be made with as much understanding as possible on the part of both the doctor and the patient. So here is some information that can help you understand the limits of healthcare science and make better decisions—as long as you realize that this is, in fact, only a *little* information from the vast amount that is available.

Patient-Based Research

While medications are initially developed in laboratories and tested using laboratory equipment and, in some cases, animals, they must eventually be tried in human beings before they can be approved for use by people. The number of people on whom they can be tried is limited by factors involving both cost and time, and the nature of the information obtained through this sort of research is therefore limited as well. So even after a drug is approved, manufacturers are required to maintain records of its effects in everyday, real-world medical use.

There is a hierarchy of research that it is useful for patients to know, because the way in which information is obtained reflects directly on its reliability. The jargon can be confusing for non-scientists—what exactly do "randomized" and "double-blind" mean, for example?

Even after a drug is approved, manufacturers are required to maintain records of its effects in everyday, real-world medical use.

Patient-Based Research Methods

1) **Anecdotal:** This simply means an observation, perhaps by only one doctor treating one patient—the doctor might report that Joan Smith had nausea and diarrhea after using a particular drug for one week.

2) **Retrospective:** This type of study collects data about events that have already happened, for example by asking people to write down how much coffee they drank every day for the past month.

3) **Prospective:** The opposite of retrospective—all data are collected after the study is designed.

4) **Clinician-assigned:** Two or more treatments are being investigated. The doctor picks which one each patient will receive.

5) **Randomized:** Again, two or more treatments are under study. But here, each patient in the study is randomly assigned to a therapy.

6) **Controlled:** Again, more than one therapy is under investigation. Generally, the treatment in question, such as a new drug, is compared to another treatment, such as a placebo, which is a sugar pill that has no true physical effect, or to the established standard of care, such as a drug already approved for a condition, or both.

7) **Double-blind:** This is the "gold standard" of medical research. It is a study in which no participant—patient or researcher—knows who is receiving which therapy. That is, patient and scientist alike are "blind" to the therapy being administered—which means not knowing who is getting, say, a new medication, and who is receiving a placebo. Double-blind studies are the least susceptible to bias and are therefore considered the best research possible.

It is perfectly reasonable to wonder, if double-blind studies are so highly regarded, why they are not the only ones done. There are a number of reasons.

No research study is wholly free of bias.

For one thing, a double-blind study is easy to do in some cases—when administering pills, for example. But it is virtually impossible in others, as when comparing types of surgical procedures. Also, although double-blind studies yield the most reliable research, they are more difficult to run than any other study type and far more expensive.

It is also worth pointing out that no study, not even a double-blind one, is wholly free of bias. The reason is that the patients included in—and excluded from—the study represent bias of a sort. For example, the vast majority of studies exclude children and pregnant women. There are perfectly sound reasons for this—the desire not to endanger young people and the unborn, the impossibility from a legal standpoint of obtaining informed consent from a minor, and so on. But this means that certain people for whom a new treatment might be highly beneficial—or highly dangerous—are systematically excluded from studies that would show the benefit or danger. Therefore, such risk or benefit will be discovered only after a treatment is accepted and its use is expanded beyond that for which it is initially approved—for example, through off-label use.

And there are more-subtle biases in patient selection as well: people above a certain age may be excluded, or people below a certain age. Also, people with certain illnesses may be left out—for example, tests of a new drug for cardiac insufficiency may systematically exclude patients with type 2 diabetes, unless the drug is specifically being tested to determine whether it improves the cardiovascular condition of diabetics.

Knowing the inherent limitations of medical research goes a long way toward helping patients understand why there is nothing simple, straightforward or universally applicable in prescribing treatments for diseases or chronic conditions.

The "Ask Your Doctor" Notion

Just about every organization, every advertisement, every source of medical information on statins, cardio-

If your doctor recommends that you start on a statin, be sure he/she knows your full medical history. vascular disease and health in general tells you to "ask your doctor." This would be easier, and would seem less like legalese, if they explained *what* to ask.

It *is* important to talk with your doctor about your personal cardiovascular risk profile and the choices available to you in defense of your own health—choices that include both lifestyle adaptations and medications such as statins. It is helpful to prepare questions in advance of your appointment with your doctor.

Questions to Ask Your Doctor

- What are my risk factors for cardiovascular disease?

- What lifestyle changes might reduce my risk enough so I will not need to take medicine for the rest of my life?

- What specific foods should I eliminate from my diet? Eat less often? In smaller portions?

- What foods should I add to my diet? In what quantities? What should I eat more often or in larger portions?

- How much and what type of exercise would you recommend, considering my age and general health?

- What medical issues or family history that would limit my type, intensity or frequency of exercise?

If your doctor recommends that you start on a statin, be sure he or she knows your full medical history, including all prescription medications you take, plus any over-the-counter medicines and any herbal or other supplements. Discuss any problems you have ever been told about regarding your liver, such as hepatitis or abnormal liver-enzyme tests, and say how much alcohol you consume weekly.

Questions to Ask About Statins

- Why are you recommending this statin? Why at this dosage?
- What specific cholesterol goals does this statin help me reach? How?
- When and why would you change the medication or the dose?
- What symptoms should I watch for and report to you?
- What are the most-common side effects with this particular statin?
- WHen is liver enzymes monitoring needed? How often?
- What if I experience side effects from taking this statin?
- How can I reduce side effects? Will side effects go away?

You will not necessarily need to ask all or even most of these questions—your doctor may provide much of the information without being asked. But it makes sense to write down any questions you consider relevant and bring them along, so that if your doctor does not address one or more of your concerns, you have a written reminder to yourself to ask about them—and straight-forward words in which to pose the question.

Questions to Ask About Side Effects

- Will this side effect go away? How long?

- Can adjusting my dose to eliminate the side effect? If so, how will that affect my cholorestrol level?

- Are there other statins that are less likely to produce this side effect? If so, can you switch me to one of those?

- Does the side effect pose a potential health risk—beyond the discomfort? If so, what do you would you recommend?

Of course, you should ask additional questions reflect-ing your personal situation. And if you are worried by some of the things you have heard about statins, say so. Your psychological comfort with the medications is an important element of your health—you need to be will-ing to take them, possibly for the rest of your life, with a feeling of comfort in using them and in their efficacy.

Tests for Cardiovascular Health

There are many tests that doctors can use to evaluate your heart health, both before you make lifestyle chang-es or begin taking statins—if they are indicated—and while you are modifying your diet and activities and taking prescribed medications. Not all doctors order all these tests for all patients—some are appropriate only under certain conditions.

There may be primary and some secondary ones for special circumstances, and it can help to know what they are and what values doctors hope to see in the test results. The farther from the normative values you are, the more likely it is that you will need to take statins and/or other medicines to bring the results into a range considered to be best for your continuing cardiac health.

Additional Tests

- **Total cholesterol, HDL, LDL, and triglycerides.** These are the basic measurements. Doctors look for total cholesterol under 200; HDL over 60; LDL under 100—some doctors prefer to see it under 80; and triglycerides under 100. These tests include ratios of certain components to others. The ratio of total cholesterol to HDL should be no more than 3.0, and the ratio of triglycerides to HDL should be no greater than 4.0.

- **Cardio C-reactive protein.** This is a marker of inflammation in the body that contributes to overall cardiovascular risk. The normal CRP level varies by lab.

- **Glucose Insulin Tolerance Test.** Measurements of fasting and one- and two-hour levels of both glucose and insulin help identify pre-diabetes or even diabetes—a significant cardiovascular risk factor. Many doctors check blood sugar but not insulin; getting data on both provides better clinical information.

- **Hemoglobin A1c—glycated hemoglobin.** Measures average blood sugar level over the previous 6 to 12 weeks. Result should be 5.6% or less; levels of 5.7% to 6.4% indicate increased diabetes risk; levels of 6.5% or higher indicate diabetes.

- **Homocysteine.** This is a measurement of folate; high levels have been linked to cardiovascular disease, although lowering the levels does not seem to help prevent cardiac problems.

- **Lipoprotein (a),** another factor that can promote the risk of heart disease, especially in men, may be relevant when LDL is elevated; normal levels vary by race and ethnicity.

- **Fibrinogen, a liver protein,** helps blood clots form. Normal range is 200 to 400 milligrams per deciliter (mg/dL).

- **Lipid peroxides or TBARS**—thiobarbituric acid reactive substances—assay is a way of determining how much oxidized cholesterol is in the body. It measures the amount of damage done by oxidative stress—a cardiovascular-disease risk factor.

Your doctor may order a variety of other tests, some more common than others, depending on your personal and family cardiac history and other factors. For example, a number of genes regulate cholesterol and metabolism, such as Apo E genes and the cholesterol ester transfer protein gene; thus, genetic testing may be part of a thorough cardiovascular workup.

The NMR LipoProfile test, from a company called LipoScience, uses an MRI—magnetic resonance imaging—scan to examine cholesterol and find out the size of the particles—it can be important in determining whether you have a considerable number of small, dense and therefore dangerous particles, or more of the light, fluffy and essentially harmless ones. And a computed tomography (CT) or electron beam computed tomography (EBT) scan of your heart can be used to evaluate overall plaque burden and calcium score. This test looks for calcium in the heart's arteries and can detect heart problems earlier than other tests do; a score higher than 100 is considered cause for concern, and a score higher than 400 indicates severe risk of cardiovascular disease. However, the test is not universally accepted and can generate false-positive readings.

This is by no means a comprehensive list of cardiovascular tests, but it would still be highly unusual for a doctor to order all of these all the time. The basic blood test for total cholesterol, HDL, LDL and triglycerides, often called a lipid panel, gives accurate and useful information and is often all that is needed to decide on a plan of action for *It would be highly unusual for a doctor to order all available tests all the time.* cardiovascular health. Other tests may be used to pin down areas of specific concern.

The message for patients is to know that there are many tests for cardiac health available, and it is perfectly reasonable to ask your doctor why he or she is ordering certain specific ones. The more you understand about what is being done and why—and what the meanings of the test results are—the more comfortable you will be in going along with your doctor's recommendations for your cardiac health, whether they involve lifestyle changes, the use of statins or other drugs, or a combination.

Bibliography & References

Begley, Sharon, "The Cholesterol Conundrum." *Saturday Evening Post*. http://www.saturdayeveningpost. com/2012/04/24/wellness/cholesterol-conundrum.html, May/June 2012.

Benji, Shamir, "Statins and Muscle Injury." http://www. empowher.com, April 28, 2012.

Braunstein, Glenn D., MD, "Be Smart on Statins: Heart Health Can't Rely on Just Cholesterol-Cutting Drugs." http://www.huffingtonpost.com/glenn-d-braunstein-md/ cholesterol-drugs_b_1405975.html, April 16, 2012.

Brice, Makini, "Good News: Americans' Average Cholesterol Levels Have Declined." http://www.medicaldaily.com/ articles/12744/20121017/good-news-americans-average-cholesterol-levels-declined.htm#DK0ploriT1Y6whP5.99, October 17, 2012.

"Can It Get Much Worse? Drug Company Now Claims Statins Recommended for Swine Flu." http://articles. mercola.com/sites/articles/archive/2009/11/28/can-it-get-much-worse--drug-company-now-claims-statins-recommended-for-swine-flu.aspx, November 28, 2009.

Carroll, Margaret D., MSPH, *et al.*, "Cholesterol Levels Improving Among U.S. Adults." JAMA 2012;308[15]:1545-1554, http://media.jamanetwork.com/news-item/cholesterol-levels-improving-among-u-s-adults/, October 17, 2012.

de Ferranti, Sarah D., MD, MPH, "Declining Cholesterol Levels in US Youths: A Reason for Optimism." *JAMA*. 2012;308(6):621-622, http://jama.jamanetwork.com/article.aspx?articleid=1309158, August 8, 2012.

"Dueling viewpoints: Should a healthy middle-aged man with elevated cholesterol take a statin drug?" *HealthNews-Review.org.* http://www.healthnewsreview.org/2012/04/dueling-viewpoints-should-a-healthy-middle-aged-man-with-elevated-cholesterol-take-a-statin-drug/, April 13, 2012.

"FDA Drug Safety Communication: Ongoing safety review of high-dose Zocor (simvastatin) and increased risk of muscle injury." http://www.fda.gov/Drugs/DrugSafety/PostmarketDrugSafetyInformationforPatientsandProviders/ucm204882.htm, March 19, 2010.

Gillinov, Marc, MD, and Steven Nissen, MD, *Heart 411: The Only Guide to Heart Health You'll Ever Need.* New York: Three Rivers Press, January 2012.

Golomb, Beatrice A., MD, PhD, *et al.*, "Effects of Statins on Energy and Fatigue with Exertion: Results from a Randomized Controlled Trial." *JAMA Internal Medicine*, Vol. 172, No. 15. http://archinte.jamanetwork.com/article.aspx?articleid=1183454, August 13/27, 2012.

Haiken, Melanie, "The Latest Statin Scare: Are You At Risk?" Forbes, February 29, 2012.

Harding, Anne, "Heart failure may worsen with statins, study says." http://www.cnn.com/2009/HEALTH/11/05/statins.heart.failure/index.html,November 5, 2009.

Huffman, Taylor, MD, et al., "Statins for the primary prevention of cardiovascular disease." *Cochrane Library.* http://summaries.cochrane.org/CD004816/statins-for-the-primary-prevention-of-cardiovascular-disease, January 31, 2013.

Hyman, Mark, MD, "Why Cholesterol May Not Be the Cause of Heart Disease." http://www.huffingtonpost.com/dr-mark-hyman/why-cholesterol-may-not-b_b_290687.html, September 20, 2009.

Isaacs, Tony, "FDA mandates new safety warnings for statin drugs due to risks of memory loss, diabetes and muscle pain." http://www.naturalnews.com/035131_statin_drugs_safety_warnings_muscle_pain.html#ixzz2LqYnRaJ2, March 3, 2012.

Japsen, Bruce, "Doctors rethinking prescribing Abbott's Niaspan: National Institutes of Health's study suggests minimal benefit, and some risk, to combining HDL cholesterol-raising drug with LDL-lowering statins." http://articles.chicagotribune.com/2011-05-31/business/ct-biz-0531-abbott-cholesterol-20110531_1_statins-ldl-lowering-stroke-risk, May 31, 2011.

Kotz, Deborah, "Increased diabetes risks from statins outweighed by heart benefits." http://www.boston.com/dailydose/2012/08/09/increased-diabetes-risks-from-statins-outweighed-heart-benefits-boston-researchers-find/ikAtz5tc2hITGb7HLnNmjN/story.html, August 9, 2012.

"Niacin and Cholesterol," UC Berkeley Wellness Letter. http://www.berkeleywellness.com/supplements/vitamins/article/niacin-and-cholesterol, February 24, 2013.

Nielsen, Sune F., PhD, Børge G. Nordestgaard, MD, DMSc, and Stig E. Bojesen, MD, PhD, DMSc, "Statin Use and Reduced Cancer-Related Mortality." New England Journal of Medicine 2012; 367:1792-1802. http://www.nejm.org/doi/full/10.1056/NEJMoa1201735, November 8, 2012.

Pierson, Ransdell, "Merck cholesterol drug fails; risks seen." http://www.reuters.com/article/2012/12/20/us-merck-cholesterol-idUSBRE8BJ0RU20121220, December 20, 2012.

Pittman, David, "FDA OKs Drug for Rare Lipid Disorder." http://www.medpagetoday.com/Cardiology/Dyslipidemia/36623, December 26, 2012.

Pollack, Andrew, "New Drugs for Lipids Set Off Race." http://www.nytimes.com/2012/11/06/business/new-drugs-for-lipids-set-off-race.html?_r=0, November 6, 2012.

Redberg, Rita F., MD, and Mitchell H. Katz, MD, "Reassessing Benefits and Risks of Statins." *New England Journal of Medicine.* http://www.nejm.org/doi/full/10.1056/NEJMc1207079, August 23, 2012.

"Rhabdomyolysis Symptoms, Causes, Treatment." http://www.medicinenet.com/rhabdomyolysis/page2.htm

Ridker, Paul M., MD, *et al.*, "Cardiovascular benefits anddiabetes risks of statin therapy in primary prevention: an analysis from the JUPITER trial." *The Lancet,* vol. 380, issue 9841, August 11, 2012.

"Risk Assessment Tool for Estimating Your 10-year Risk of Having a Heart Attack." http://hp2010.nhlbihin.net/atpiii/calculator.asp

Seneff, Stephanie, "Statins and Myoglobin: How Muscle Pain and Weakness Progress to Heart, Lung and Kidney Failure." http://people.csail.mit.edu/seneff/statins_muscle_damage_heart_failure.html

"Should Healthy People Take Cholesterol Drugs to Prevent Heart Disease?" *Wall Street Journal,* http://online.wsj.com/article/SB1000142405297020347100457714505356618569.4.html, January 23, 2012.

Sifferlin, Alexandra, "Should You Take Statins? Study Says Heart Benefits Outweigh Diabetes Risk.".http://healthland.time.com/2012/08/10/should-you-take-statins-study-says-heart-benefits-outweigh-diabetes-risk/#ixzz2LqZm75if, August 10, 2012.

"Statin Adverse Effects: Statin Effects Study, University of California at San Diego." *Clinical Medicine and Research,* 10(3): 158. https://www.statineffects.com/info/adverse_effects.htm, August 2012.

"Statin Medications and Heart Disease." The Cleveland Clinic. http://my.clevelandclinic.org/heart/prevention/cholesterol/statin-medications-and-heart-disease.aspx

"Statins Are Not Equally Beneficial for Thromboembolic and Heart Disease."*Pulmonary Reviews*. http://www.pulmonaryreviews.com/Article.aspx?ArticleId=WUnYjy0c6s4=, 2009;14(12):13-15.

"Statins: Are these cholesterol-lowering drugs right for you?" The Mayo Clinic. http://www.mayoclinic.com/health/statins/CL00010

"Statins may be linked to cancer survival." http://www.reuters.com/article/2012/11/07/us-statins-cancer-idUSBRE-8A62H020121107

Stengler, Mark, NMD, "Statin Sensationalism." http://blog.markstengler.com/statin-sensationalism/, November 28, 2012.

Stengler, Mark, NMD, "Statin Use Linked to Diabetes." http://blog.markstengler.com/statin-use-linked-to-diabetes/, January 17, 2013.

"The Use of Administrative Data and Natural Language Processing to Estimate the Incidence of Statin-related Rhabdomyolysis." http://www.ncbi.nlm.nih.gov/pmc/articles/PMC3421398/

Van De Graaff, Eric, MD, "Statins for heart disease and stroke, and debunking statin myths." http://www.kevinmd.com/blog/2010/08/statins-heart-disease-stroke-debunking-statin-myths.html, August 27, 2010.

Wehrwein, Peter, "Statin use is up, cholesterol levels are down: Are Americans' hearts benefiting? " http://www.health.harvard.edu/blog/statin-use-is-up-cholesterol-levels-are-down-are-americans-hearts-benefiting-201104151518, April 15, 2011.

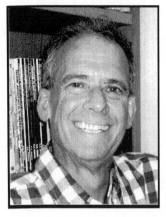

Mark J. Estren, Ph.D., received doctorates in psychology and in English from the University at Buffalo and a master's degree in journalism from Columbia University.

A Pulitzer-winning journalist, Dr. Estren has held top-level positions at numerous print and broadcast news organizations for more than 30 years, ranging from producer of "Report on Medicine" for CBS Radio to frequent health-related reporting for the *Bottom Line* newsletter group. Other affiliations include *The Washington Post, Miami Herald, Philadelphia Inquirer*, United Press International, and CBS and ABC News. He was named one of *Fortune* magazine's "People to Watch."

Experienced in business as well as health and medicine, Dr. Estren was general manager of Financial News Network, creator and executive producer of the national edition *of The Nightly Business Report*, and editor of *High Technology Business* magazine. Dr. Estren's offices are in Fort Myers, Florida. His site is markjestren.com. Please visit.

RONIN BOOKS FOR INDEPENDENT MINDS